Room 105

Readers' Lives Are Touched
Through Reading *Room 105:*

"I read the manuscript of *Room 105* prior to undergoing life-threatening surgery. I am not a reader, generally; nevertheless, I could not put this book down. Through it, I discovered a loving God, whom I could know personally."

> —Kathy Szydlak, who has a potentially fatal heart condition

"Marcus' son Andrew and my son Glenn both had brain tumors; they were in the hospital together. When Marcus shared his story with me, I was horrified to learn that he had lost his wife to cancer, and was likely to lose his son, too...I asked myself, *How could this man possibly believe that God was not to blame—and that such a God really loves us?* Here he was, amidst such terrible tragedy, watching, along with me, our children literally dying before our very eyes, yet he was full of hope, faith and a serenity that came from who-knows-where! There was not even a hint of the anger, self-pity or hopelessness that the rest of us were feeling at various times.

"At the time, I chalked him up as either a 'God nut,' a sham, or just someone gone insane due to the stress of it all. How wrong I was!

"The more I watched Marcus, the more I realized that he had something I didn't—a calmness, an undergirding love for God and his fellowman that seemed to help him cope, no matter how depressing that day's report from the doctor was. And I could see it in the children, too: Andrew telling Glenn, 'Jesus loves you' and meaning it; Glenn nodding in a deep, knowing way, accepting it, not cringing, like I did. I decided that I wanted what Marcus and the boys had.

"Marcus knew that I was angry with God, wondering if He indeed existed at all. Marcus mailed me portions of his manuscript, in the hope that they might help me. That's when this man touched my heart. I suddenly knew what he and the boys knew: that God did really love me—with a love of indescribable magnitude.

"Without this man and his book, it is doubtful whether I would even be alive today; in the heartbreaking devastation and desperation caused by my son's death, I could easily have taken my life. Marcus has become someone very special to me; God has used him in my life. I like to think of Marcus as my very own guardian angel, sent from my gracious heavenly Father, at the exact time I needed him. Perhaps Andrew was the same for Glenn.

"May Marcus' book touch your life as it has touched mine. Enjoy!"

—**Rhonda Smith**, who lost her son to cancer

"When our God could have prevented it, but didn't; when the very One to whom we could run seemed to have betrayed us; then what? Marcus has been to the place 'where deep calls unto deep.' In this book there is life for those who have been to that place."

—**Jean Lagettie**, mother of two children killed in a car accident

"This book records for us the travel of one of God's redeemed families as the Truth about Jesus is incarnated in their lives. Do not expect to read this book without being touched by its drama. Having known Marcus for many years, I can heartily vouch for this journal. It describes a journey which proclaims the authentic faith that those in Christ Jesus have come to lean hard upon."

—**Rev. Don Broadwater**, minister of religion

"After reading *Room 105*, I realized that those who care for the sick, suffering and disabled...have a silent ministry. The reader of this book cannot help but be touched deeply, and will want to reassess his/her priorities in life.

"There is also a warning here: not to follow the teachings of mere men. God and His infallible Word are the only sure foundations on which to build your future."

—**Nicola (Nicky) Fox**, mother of an intellectually disabled child

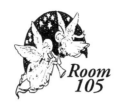

ROOM 105

The Compelling True-Life Story of Victory Over Suffering & Death

ROOM 105

The Compelling True-Life Story of Victory Over Suffering & Death

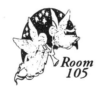

Marcus Luedi
with
Allen Roberts

MEISTER PRESS / *Charleston, South Carolina USA*

Requests for permission to reprint portions of this book may be directed to:

Marcus Luedi
PO Box 257 / Coffs Harbour / New South Wales 2450, Australia
Phone (from USA): 011-61-266-537065; (within Australia): 0266-537065
FAX (from USA): 011-61-266-526823; (within Australia): 0266-526823
E-mail: rodfox@midcoast.com.au

Published in Charleston, South Carolina, USA by Meister Press, a division of DunkMeister Communications. Unless otherwise noted, all Scripture quotations are quoted from the King James Version of the Bible. Inspiration for angel in cover design by permission of Jack T. Chick; such permission is hereby gratefully acknowledged. Although all the stories in this book are historically accurate, some names of individuals have been changed for confidentiality considerations.

For information on purchasing this book, either singly or in quantity, or for booking the author(s) to speak at your church, club, business or other organization, please contact:

Kurt & Rebecca Niederer
3021 Mountainbrook Rd. / Charlotte, NC / 28210 USA
Phone: 704/553-0239 / FAX: 704/553-7532
E-mail: swisseng@aol.com

or you may contact the author, Marcus Luedi, in Australia at the addresses listed above.

Requests for editorial and publishing services may be directed to:

Duncan Jaenicke, President, Meister Press
PO Box 1296 / Goose Creek, SC 29445 USA
Phones: (toll-free) 888/BOOK-070 or 803/824-0706
FAX: 803/824-6759 / E-mail: dunctalk@ix.netcom.com

Library of Congress Cataloging-in-Publication Data

Luedi, Marcus
Room 105 The Compelling True-Life Story of Victory
Over Suffering & Death / Marcus Luedi
p. cm.
Includes bibliographical references.
ISBN 0-9643136-2-6
1. Biography. 2. Religious—Inspirational. 3. Cancer. 4. Prayer I. Title.

Printed in the United States of America

Contents

Acknowledgements ix
Foreword xi
Prologue xiii
Chapter 1 1
Chapter 2 7
Chapter 3 15
Chapter 4 21
Chapter 5 28
Chapter 6 34
Chapter 7 38
Chapter 8 46
Chapter 9 57
Chapter 10 63
Chapter 11 69
Chapter 12 75
Chapter 13 85
Chapter 14 88
Chapter 15 95
Chapter 16 106
Chapter 17 110
Chapter 18 117
Chapter 19 128
Chapter 20 134
Chapter 21 140
Chapter 22 144
Chapter 23 151
Chapter 24 158
Chapter 25 163
Chapter 26 173
Chapter 27 177
Chapter 28 182
Chapter 29 188
Chapter 30 192
Afterword 198
End Notes 204

Room 105

Acknowledgements

We would like to thank sincerely all those persons who have provided the prayerful and practical support, without which this book could never have been written. Early on, we tried to list you all specifically, but that was terribly frustrating, since the next day we'd think of others we'd missed. Some people, who have helped us significantly, requested that they be not even mentioned.

So, we have decided it was better to thank you all anonymously. You have all shown us a warm spirit of friendship, and have been a crucial part of this story becoming a book.

You all know who you are, and God knows. And with that, we are satisfied.

Room 105

Foreword

Ifirst met Marcus Luedi in 1969, shortly after he and his family migrated to Australia. My wife Faye and I became close friends with Marianne and Marcus, and soon there was a strong spiritual bond between our two families.

Marcus and I not only worshiped together in the same church, but also studied the Bible and prayed together in my home, along with some other deeply committed Christian men. This dynamic prayer support group continued for almost two decades and still meets today. It has become a crucially important lifeline for each of us, not only in our personal lives, but also in our work and ministries.

Without the spiritual support of Marcus and these other godly men, I know I could not have faced and dealt with the many challenges that have confronted me in local government and as Mayor of this city.

So close were the ties between us that Marcus and his family became an integral part of our lives. In addition to having worshiped with them, we also have rejoiced with them in times of happiness, and wept with them in times of suffering and grief. Being able to stand alongside this precious family as they experienced potentially devastating sickness and loss—first of a wife and mother, then of an only son—was not a burden for us but rather a privilege.

We were blessed and encouraged as, by God's enablement, Marcus bore nobly the stresses and pressures God allowed him to experience. Through several years of excruciating affliction, Marcus continued to show his love for Jesus, and his absolute trust in God and His Word.

His example has been an inspiration to many. May this book reveal his example to many more.

John B. Smith
Mayor, City of Coffs Harbour
New South Wales, Australia

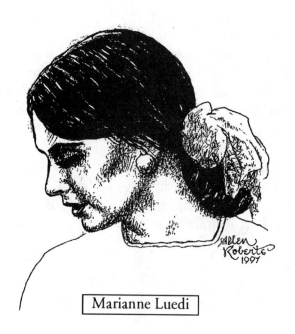

Marianne Luedi

Room 105

Prologue

"Mr. Luedi, your wife has just passed away. I'm sorry." The words numbed me. I sat at my desk, motionless, without feeling, for the next 10 minutes in the dark early morning silence of my study.

I couldn't accept that God had let me down after I had put my faith in Him over these last six months. Even though Marianne's health had deteriorated rapidly, during the last three weeks of this period, I had earnestly sought to stand on God's Word and His promises. I was actually certain that Marianne would be healed and would not even talk with her about the possibility of her dying. Though Dr. Scott had informed me that Marianne had only three weeks to live, I still expected that God would perform a miracle. Certainly no one had exercised more faith than I. So why wouldn't God honor my unshakable trust in Him?

Suddenly I remembered that I was expected at the hospital. My two younger children—Natasha, my 13-year-old daughter, and Andrew, my eight-year-old son, who was still recovering from a brain tumor operation—were still sound asleep. It was a typical crisp autumn morning, still dark on March 12, 1988, when I arrived at Baringa Private Hospital in Coffs Harbour. Dr. Scott had waited there for me. With a few brief words, he guided me into the room where the body of my once so beautiful wife was lying. He left me alone there.

I whispered a prayer as I sat at Marianne's bedside. I kissed her gently on the forehead. Somehow I could not accept God's dealings in all this. The questions began to come. They were cynical and angry.

Why, God, why have You let me down? Why haven't You honored my faith? Can I ever trust You again? Something must have gone terribly wrong! You must do something! I can never stand in a pulpit and preach on the subject of faith again. I just can't understand You anymore.

For the next few minutes, as I sat at the bedside, our 23 years of highly eventful, often turbulent marriage, passed before me. How quickly they had flown by! Marianne was only 47 years old. This was far younger than the expected biblical life-span of 70 years. She was too young to leave this earth! Natasha now needed her mother at the beginning of her tender teenage years. Andrew, particularly, who still had a long way to go in his recovery, needed his mother.

What an exceptionally beautiful young lady Marianne had been when we first met! How cruel that terrible enemy called cancer.

My thoughts went back to the time when we had first met. I was already over 30 years of age and still a bachelor with a promising future in business. Even though I had grown up in the Evangelical Brotherhood Church, a very fundamental denomination in Switzerland, I had come to the point in my life where I decided I didn't need God any more. Life was too challenging and fascinating without the limitations of church rules and regulations which fettered me. I had the world at my feet. I didn't even believe in marriage. In fact, I pitied my younger brother and sister when they made their marriage vows before God. Yet deep down I felt an inner emptiness and I tried to compensate for these feelings by traveling the world. This did not satisfy me. Nor did fulfillment come from the many relationships I'd had with women—until I met Marianne. From that moment I had wanted to marry her. Suddenly, marriage, which for me had never been important, was ironically now all important. I sensed that the emptiness I felt would disappear forever if I should marry Marianne.

She had just been awarded a four-year diploma in acting. Young girls in the acting profession often do modeling to survive. For aspiring film actresses, the opportunity of landing that lucrative major role in the movies is very rare and many have to undertake a second job to earn their living in the meantime. Marianne did this and applied for a secretary's position in the firm where I worked. On the day I first met her, I was enchanted by her striking beauty and soon we were going out together. I learned that she'd had a Catholic upbringing, but religion didn't worry either of us. When Marianne realized that our relationship had become serious, she confessed to me that she was the unmarried mother of a 10-month-old baby girl named Claudia. Here was a challenge! Was my love for Marianne so deep that I could accept her daughter as well, or was I interested only in Marianne—this lovely woman who had so infatuated me?

My love was indeed real and I accepted them both. What impressed me most was the fact that Marianne hadn't had an abortion, as many of her friends had encouraged her to do. Deep down there were clearly some moral values still alive from her religious upbringing, even though at that time she did not have a personal relationship with God.

At the time of our engagement my company promoted me to an important position in Paris, to liaise between the Headquarters in Zurich and their newly acquired firm in France. The date for our marriage had to be arranged quickly and for the first time in many years I spoke to my parents about my future plans, my bride, and my work. Having been aware of my parents' strict fundamental Bible beliefs, I was prepared for strong opposition, so planned a compromise which I hoped would be acceptable to both sets of parents. We decided to baptize our future children in the Catholic faith to please Marianne's parents, and so as not to hurt my parents, we planned our wedding in a Protestant Church.

This arrangement seemed acceptable to all parties. And how delighted I was to be marrying the most stunning young lady in Zurich. Marianne's beauty, her outgoing and happy nature, her sparkling eyes and bubbling laughter, captivated virtually everyone who met her. I knew that all my colleagues envied me. However, the big question was, how would a young woman with such obvious sex appeal fit into my strict conservative family?

I will never forget the Saturday afternoon when I finally introduced her to my parents. Marianne was dressed, as she normally was, in a mini-skirt with high-heeled shoes. She wore glittering bracelets, ear rings and her usual make-up. I imagined that my parents would be angry that I had chosen such a modern young lady, and was ready for war. I was in fact determined to disown them both if I detected any rejection of my bride. But to my surprise we were given a hearty welcome and my mother cooked us my favorite meal. I hadn't expected such royal treatment. We stayed for the night and, the next morning, I was astonished to see my mother polishing Marianne's shoes. That action spoke more than a sermon to me.

The wedding was arranged for March 26, 1966 and it was on this occasion that my parents met Marianne's family for the first time. I was relieved that everything went so well. One big step was behind us. Marianne and I spent our honeymoon on the Isola Bella in Italy and a few days later flew to Paris. At last our new life together had begun.

Although Marianne and I had married on the understanding that our relationship would last, I sensed that both Marianne's and my parents had doubts that it would. I was later to discover that all four of them had prayed that God would somehow keep us together.

As I pondered our past two decades, the door in the hospital room quietly opened. It was Dr. Scott. Brutally, I was thrown back to reality. No, I wasn't dreaming. My heart ached. Marianne was gone. Marianne was dead! Why had God taken Marianne from us?

Dr. Scott knew how I felt. There was not much to be said. He accompanied me to the car and I drove home, sad in my heart, my head full of those seemingly unanswerable questions. But I had to be brave because my children needed me, now more than ever before.

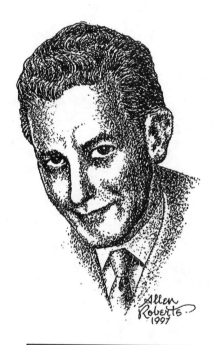

Marcus Luedi as a young man.

Room 105

Chapter 1

As I was introduced to my first bouillabaisse (a sort of fish soup) at the restaurant Chez Loury, I wasn't aware I was dining in one of the world's most famous seafood restaurants. What did it matter, anyhow? My firm could afford it.

I had been on a business trip for over two weeks and had left my wife and our two-year-old daughter Claudia alone in Paris. How were they getting on? I couldn't contact them because, just weeks before my trip around France, we had moved into a two-bedroom apartment near the Eiffel Tower, and the phone had not yet been installed. So each day I sent a postcard to my wife, but because I was constantly on the move, she couldn't contact me. I missed my family.

My head office in Zurich had bought out one of the biggest central-heating companies in France. Our Swiss product, which was far more sophisticated and modern, had to be introduced onto the French market. I needed to know the existing distributors, the mentality of the French business people and the market possibilities. I traveled with a Swiss engineer. It was certainly a great opportunity to get to know the countryside, the people—and the food.

Marseille was the halfway point of our trip. From the Mediterranean port we still had to travel through central France to the Atlantic coast and then back to Paris. Throughout our trip we had dined on the finest food and wine; twice a day for three weeks. But all I wanted was the simple potato salad Marianne would prepare for me in our home. I wrote to her saying I planned to arrive in two days.

I requested that she not make a big celebration feast, but simply prepare a potato salad!

****

It was so good to be back with my young family. After reading through all the mail which had accumulated during my absence, Marianne said she had a surprise for me. What could it be? She held a letter in her hands. It was addressed to her. Her manner was a little strange as she handed it over to me. Her eyes were fixed on me to see my reaction. I couldn't believe what I was reading and read it again, this time aloud. "You are invited to play a role in our next James Bond film." What more could she want? This was her chance for a breakthrough.

After all, she had so far played only small movie roles. "Marianne," I exclaimed, "this is the chance of your life!"

"But I would have to be away from you and Claudia for months!" she responded.

"Oh, darling," I said, "it doesn't matter. I will support you. You know what it means to play in a James Bond film? What an opportunity! The movie will be filmed in the Bernese Mountains in Switzerland. When you are working there, your parents can look after Claudia. I can't see any problems."

So far, I had seen Marianne in some of her film roles and on TV commercials here and there. Currently there was a campaign by a fashion company who used Marianne as a model. A large picture of her was displayed at every Metro station in Paris. How proud I was to see my wife's face every time I went down the steps to the underground. Marianne's picture was there for about a month. But the James Bond film would open up a career for life!

I said this to her as I hugged her in excitement. She was silent in my arms. "You must accept this offer darling," I whispered insistently.

Still she said nothing.

Then gently she withdrew from my embrace. She took both my hands in hers and looked steadily into my eyes. "Marcus," she said, almost sternly, "I am married now."

With that, she took the letter from my hand and, holding me in her gaze, tore it slowly and deliberately into pieces.

Marianne knew very well what she had done and, humanly speaking, why she had done it at that time. However, in retrospect, we came to understand that God, through that decision, was preparing us both for a much higher vocation—a spiritual ministry that we could never have imagined.

The proprietor of our enterprise came to Paris and spoke with me. What he said was a kind of compensation for Marianne's rejection of the opportunity to become famous. He said that the next promotion for me would be to Regional Manager. The future looked bright. On October 4, 1966, our second daughter was born. We gave her the name Sandra Patricia. At that time it was my aim to reach the top in my career.

Even though neither Marianne nor I was a practicing Christian, we thought it appropriate to baptize our new baby. The opportunity was given to us to baptize Sandra in Notre Dame Cathedral. After all, Marianne's religion was Roman Catholic. Both Marianne and I had purposely denied what little faith we did have from childhood, because we felt too restricted by its teachings and wanted to attain our own goals in life without God. For me, then, religion spiritually meant nothing, but to baptize Sandra in the Notre Dame, socially meant everything. Consequently, early in 1967, Marianne, Claudia and I, with two witnesses, presented our baby to a priest, and the celebration took place in a little corner of Notre Dame Cathedral.

The year 1967 was one of unrest. We witnessed, on TV, the six-day Israeli-Palestinian War and never in my life had I seen so many worried people. During that crisis, people were walking the streets with their earphones to hear the news, which was broadcast every half hour. After six days, the war was over and Israel started a new chapter in her young history as a nation.

The next year, I witnessed even greater unrest, this time in France itself, especially among the communist unions. This escalated into a general strike. A million people marched with banners along the Champs Élysées. Within a few days the shelves of the supermarkets were empty. There was no garbage collection, no taxis, no trains or even planes flying. Everything stood still. Every day the situation grew more serious. The tanks in the Bois de Boulogne were already in position. Would there be civil war? It was reported that President De Gaulle had left by helicopter—probably for Germany to arrange talks with the French Army stationed there with the allies.

The French franc lost so much of its value that no foreign bank was willing to accept it. Businesses were suffering badly. Our French branch never recovered financially from this situation. Things looked very bad. Our future seemed so uncertain that Marianne, unbeknown to me, started to read a Bible that my mother had given me for my 30th birthday. Neither of us had desired to read the Bible before this. One day at 3:30 a.m., Marianne woke me up, very fearful.

"What's the matter, darling?" I asked.

"Listen Marcus, and please don't laugh, but I have a very serious question."

"What is it?" I asked, my eyes barely open.

"If you were to die today, where would you go?" she asked. "To Heaven or Hell?"

What a curious question at 3:30 in the morning! I shook my head in unbelief, but sensing Marianne's seriousness, I answered, "To be perfectly frank, I would go straight to Hell."

"What!" she exclaimed in unbelief. "Why don't you change your life then, if you know that so clearly? I hope to go to Heaven."

"Change my life? No thank you!" I replied. "The Christian life is too hard! I tried it when I was 16 but I realized that I could not live like St. Paul. It is impossible for a young man in a world surrounded by all sorts of temptations. And, after all, I am happy the way I am. Why should I change? I am not the only person heading for Hell. I will have plenty of good company there. Please, Marianne—let me sleep. I have a busy day in front of me."

Because of the deteriorating economic climate, the proprietor who had recently promised me promotion, found it necessary to come frequently to Paris. He was a very personable gentleman in his 60s. He would often visit us in our home. I was somewhat flattered that he spent so much time with us and showed such interest in us as a family.

One evening he invited Marianne and me to go with him to a nightclub. The champagne flowed freely throughout the entire evening and on into the early hours of the morning. At about 2:00 a.m. he suggested we go to his hotel room. On our arrival there he offered us a large range of the finest French brandy. It was then that I began to see him in a new light. The more he drank, the more he began to lose his gentlemanly manners. His inhibitions began to fall away. He told Marianne to call him Walter. Such a practice was very unusual in European circles. He did not extend the same invitation to me and this concerned me.

The next day at work he asked me a question. "Mr. Luedi, would you mind if Marianne met me tomorrow in the Champs Élysées? I have to buy some presents before I leave for Zurich. I need a woman's advice."

"No problem," I replied, "I'm sure Marianne would be happy to help you make some suitable choices." Marianne arranged for baby-sitters and the next day he called for her in his chauffeur-driven limousine. She spent the afternoon with him.

When I returned from work that day, Marianne was obviously very agitated.

"What's wrong?" I asked.

"Never," she said with disgust, "never let me be alone with your boss again!"

"Why, what happened?" I asked, puzzled.

"I've had the most awful day," she said. "Walter asked me to marry him. He pleaded with me and told me he would divorce his wife if I would agree to marry him."

I was deeply shocked by this. There could never again be any trust between my boss and the two of us. I knew that Marianne would have strongly rebuffed this man's scurrilous proposition and as a result my future in the firm would now be in jeopardy.

Although I recoiled from the prospect of ever even seeing my boss again, I resolved to go to work the next day as I normally would do. We met in his office. He was about to leave for Zurich and, as he shook my hand, I saw a load of embarrassment and guilt in his face. He left quickly.

It was not long after this that I started getting signals that I had no future prospects in the business. Although I had given many years of devoted service there, it soon became quite clear that my executive career was virtually over. There was no purpose in my staying with the company. So I resolved to leave. I had no idea what I would do or where we would go.

I was completely disillusioned, with no plans or prospects. For the first time in my life, I was the victim of circumstances over which I had absolutely no control. Marianne and I were both bewildered and disoriented with uncertainty.

There was only one thing of which we were certain. We both wanted to get as far away from the business world of Paris as we possibly could—even if it meant living somewhere on the other side of the world. We both needed time away and time out.

*Room
105*

Chapter 2

The opportunity for a change was about to come in a most unexpected way.

"How would you like to go to Australia, darling?" I asked.

"I'd love to go," Marianne replied. "But how could we afford it?" she asked. "With our family it would cost a fortune—and what would you do to support us when we got there? Where would we live? It all costs money."

"I don't know the answers to all your questions dear, but I guess we can try and find some out. Why don't I start by contacting the Australian Embassy?" I did this the following morning.

When I returned in the early afternoon, Marianne greeted me at our front door.

"You won't believe this, darling," I said, "but the Australian Government will provide us with free travel from here to Australia—for both of us and our children! Free travel and, believe it or not, even free accommodations for us all when we stop over in London!"

"Marcus," she said with an incredulous smile, "surely you're joking!"

"No, I'm not. It's true—and here's something else. From the day we arrive in Australia, the Australian Government will pay us a family allowance until we find guaranteed employment!"

"What do we have to do to be eligible for all this?" Marianne asked.

"All we need do is sign a statement indicating that we will stay in Australia for a minimum of two years. How would you feel about that, dear?"

"Well, I'm not sure how we'd cope with living for two years in a Third World country."

"Marianne," I laughed, "Australia is not a Third World country; look at these brochures. See, it is a highly industrialized Western country with modern cities and excellent living conditions."

Marianne examined each brochure in delighted amazement. Then she looked up at me, with that roguish smile of hers, and said, "Marcus, let's do it. Let's all go!"

We filled out our application forms at once and within a month had successfully completed the necessary interviews and medical examinations. All we needed were our visas, and these, we were assured, would be available in six months. It now seemed certain that we would be migrating to Australia. So we sent our valuable antique furniture to Zurich where we knew we could sell it for a huge profit, then terminated our apartment lease. Having cut all our ties with France, we went to Switzerland to await the issuing of our visas.

It was here that we met a man who was to have a highly significant influence upon our lives. His name was Jack Lehman, a 63-year-old friend of my father. Jack was an unusual man. He was short of stature and wiry of build. In spite of his years, Jack was hyperactive, physically and mentally. But, for Marianne and myself, the most unusual thing about him was that his home was in Australia. He owned a beef cattle ranch there in a curiously named country town called *Woolgoolga.*

When we told him we were in the process of migrating to Australia, his face lit up. In a bizarre accent that was a mixture of Swiss German and Australian drawl, he said, "Come and stay with me in Woolgoolga! There's an empty house on my property—you can live in it rent free for as long as you like!"

I looked across at Marianne. She was visibly overwhelmed. Jack Lehman had just removed one of her major concerns—namely, a place for us all to live. But there was more.

"I'll help you settle in," he added, "get you a job if you need one, Marcus. What do you do for a living?"

"I'm a business executive." I answered.

It was obvious what Jack was thinking: *Can't see much need for one of those in Woolgoolga,* but he didn't verbalize it; instead, he simply said, "Well, Marcus, you'll just have to unsaddle the horse." I was later to find out what Jack meant by this cryptic outback comment—"unsaddle the horse."

Jack Lehman's influence went much further than the provision of accommodation and work for us in Australia. Jack, rough diamond though he was, had a deep and personal Christian belief. Although this was not important to Marianne or myself at the time, Jack's faith and his willingness to share it were eventually to exert an effect upon us that neither of us could ever have imagined.

As the time for the issuing of our visas came closer, we began to consider more carefully the implications of what we were about to do. Then, on January 24, 1969, when the visas actually arrived, we found ourselves swept along on a flood of mixed emotions.

We would be leaving our loved ones behind. Would we ever see them again? How would our family cope with a totally new culture—its people, its language, its food? Would we acclimatize to the summer heat of the Australian bush? Would the children be able to assimilate? How easily would they be able to make new Australian friends?

Then there was this compulsory two-year stay. If we broke those conditions, we would have to reimburse the Government of Australia. On the other hand, two years did seem workable. Claudia was four years old and Sandra two. During those two years we would all be able to become skilled in the nuances of the new Australian language—a matter which was very important to any future positions I might hold in business. The girls wouldn't miss any elementary school. They would start Kindergarten in Australia and be ready for higher classes when we returned. Marianne's and my parents were very sad that we were leaving them, but knowing that we would, in all probability, be back after two years made the separation a little easier.

Finally, the time for us to say good-bye to my parents had arrived. It was February 14, 1969 as we stood with them in the front garden of their house on the shore of beautiful Lake Hallwyl. This was very painful for me. My heart ached as I hugged them both. How downcast they were and yet how brave. I had the feeling that I wouldn't see them again, but tried not to show it. For Marianne it was equally difficult. Tears were shed. Marianne's father had his sunglasses on—I suspected to cover up. The next day we were standing with our two girls on Platform 12 at Zurich Central Station. Most members of our families were there. We waved to them as our train pulled out on the first leg of our journey. Geneva would be our first stop; a four hour trip. Leaving our homeland was one of the hardest experiences of our life together so far. My brother, Gideon, met us at Geneva Airport. He was the only member of our family to bid us farewell before we flew out to London.

At Heathrow Airport we met several more emigrants from Europe who, like ourselves, were destined for Australia. Like us, they were seeking new freedom and a new life.

The journey from London to Australia took some 26 hours. The flight, as we sought to manage our children, seemed interminable. Marianne and I couldn't sleep, but our two girls did. They had been marvelous so far, not a word of dissatisfaction or complaint. There was great excitement as we came in over the continent of Australia from the west. For five more hours we flew across its desert vastness. We realized, as we gazed down on it, how brown it was; it really was a sunburned country—so different from home.

Eventually, tired and tense, we touched down in Sydney. As our plane taxied towards the terminal, I noticed that all of the traffic controllers were wearing summer clothing—open-necked shirts with short sleeves. And here we all were, rugged up, in our Northern Hemisphere winter garb. I was wearing my woolen three-piece business suit. As I reached into our overhead baggage compartments, I saw my heavy fur-lined woolen overcoat. Although I'd paid a very high price for it in Switzerland, I couldn't bear the thought of even carrying it, let alone wearing it in this sweltering hot February heat. I decided to leave it in the locker. As we struggled down the steps with the rest of our belongings, someone tapped me on the shoulder. It was one of our air-hostesses.

"Excuse me, sir, but is this your overcoat? I found it folded in the compartment above where you were sitting."

"Yes, it is," I responded with a somewhat false smile. "Thank you." I took the coat and strapped it to one of our suitcases.

When the customs officials began to speak to me I was not able to answer them, because I could not follow what they were saying.

"What are they saying?" Marianne whispered from behind me when she saw I was not responding.

"I don't know," I whispered back with embarrassment. "I can't understand their questions."

"But I thought you knew English," she said out of the corner of her mouth.

"I do," I mumbled in reply, "I learned it at school. But this is different. This is Australian."

When we were cleared by Customs, we were immediately directed, along with many other fellow migrants, towards a number of waiting buses. Without ceremony, we were bundled, with our luggage, into one of these. When every seat was filled, we moved off. Marianne and I were aware that we would be required to stay for a short period in a migrant hostel before moving to our accommodation in Woolgoolga. We assumed that this hostel would be somewhere in the vicinity of Sydney. How wrong we were about this.

The bus was crowded. It had no air conditioning. The morning sun beat down mercilessly upon us as we perspired in our thick winter clothing.

Our bus traveled through the city of Sydney, then across its outer suburbs and finally into the surrounding countryside. Where was this hostel? How we longed to move into our temporary quarters there, unpack our baggage, let the children run about for a bit and then put them to bed between clean sheets.

Soon we were traveling along a major highway through undulating country.

The hills were dotted with gray-green gum trees. There was no sign of a town or even village—certainly no hostel.

An hour passed. Then another. Our two little girls were becoming increasingly uncomfortable and distressed. After a 26-hour flight, now this. We'd all had enough. I resolved to find out what was going on. I went forward to the driver.

"Excuse me," I asked, "but exactly where are we heading?"

He mumbled something that I could not understand.

"Pardon me, but what was that again?" I asked.

He repeated what he'd said. It sounded something like Bonegilla.
"Where's that?" I asked.
"It's in the state of Victoria," he replied.
"How much further is it?" I inquired.
"Oh, about 250 miles," he said casually.

Two hundred fifty miles, I thought to myself. *We couldn't be going that far, surely!*

I knew that to convert this distance into the familiar kilometers we used in Europe, I'd have to multiply 250 by 1.6. I did the calculation rapidly in my head.

Goodness me, I thought, *that's around 400 kilometers—the total distance from one end of Switzerland to the other!*

In dismay I turned and headed back up the aisle towards Marianne. She was the only woman on the bus with children. Her face was flushed with the heat.

The strain she was experiencing showed unmistakably in the lines around her mouth. Her eyes were closed, but I knew she wasn't asleep. Her arm was around Claudia, who sat awkwardly in the seat next to her near the window. Sandra lay in Marianne's lap, her blonde hair matted with perspiration on her tiny forehead.

"Let me take her, darling," I said, as I leaned across and picked Sandra up in my arms. I sat down with her in the seat behind. I wondered whether I dared tell Marianne that we still had 400 kilometers to travel.

"How far is it to the hostel?" Marianne asked in a voice that was taut with stress. Her eyes were still closed and she did not turn her head.

"Over two hundred," I answered, not specifying that this was only miles and not kilometers.

Towards mid-afternoon our driver pulled in at a roadhouse. Everyone got off the bus. Marianne, still with Sandra in her arms, stood on the footpath.

"Let's all go in and have a nice cool drink," I said as Claudia and I joined her.

Marianne said nothing. She was obviously very upset.

I put my arm around her shoulder. "Darling, I know how you feel. You'll feel better after you've had a break. Let's all go inside and have that drink."

Marianne refused to budge. "I'm not moving from this spot!" she said angrily.

"Marianne, be reasonable," I pleaded, as I tried to lead her towards the roadhouse.

"No," she snapped, "I'm staying right here and I'm certainly not getting back on that bus!" With that she turned away and stood there on the footpath with Sandra clasped to her bosom. "I'm staying here," she said, her eyes narrowing with firm determination, "and I want all our baggage here with us on this footpath!" she said emphatically, pointing down to the spot where she stood.

I realized that her endurance had been stretched to its limits. I needed to be equally firm to bring the situation back under control.

"Marianne," I said with all the authority I could muster, "you just can't stay here."

"I can and I will!" she said with equal resolution. "Tell the driver to get our suitcases off that bus and put them here on this footpath."

"Marianne," I began, "this is stupid ...."

"Tell that driver to get our cases this minute. I want them right here, right now!" she demanded.

By this time, some of the passengers were returning to the bus and saw us arguing. There seemed no way of defusing the situation while Marianne was in such an emotional state. So, to avoid further confrontation, I went into the roadhouse and told the driver to remove our baggage from the bus.

He did this without comment, then climbed back into his seat. Within a few more minutes all the other passengers were back on board. The driver revved the engine. He was ready to leave as we stood there with the children, our two large suitcases on the footpath beside us. I determined to make one final attempt to get Marianne back on the bus.

I stood directly in front of her and put both my hands firmly on her shoulders. Then, looking earnestly into her eyes, said slowly, "Darling, we can't stay here. We don't know anyone in this place. We don't even know where we are. I had no idea that it would be like this. Believe me, I do appreciate how you feel, but we just have to go on. Let's get back on that bus."

The air brakes hissed and the bus driver reached for the lever that would close the door. I picked up both our cases and dumped them in front of the baggage compartment. I went back to Marianne and the children. I put my arm around Marianne's waist and gently led her back to the bus. The drama was over. We boarded without comment and returned to our seats where we sat in exhausted silence. There seemed to be nothing left for either of us to say.

It was almost nightfall when we arrived at Bonegilla. By this time, the jet lag of our long flight and our emotionally harrowing bus journey had reduced us all to an almost zombie-like state. All we wanted to do was collapse into a bed and sleep solidly for two days. But this day was not yet over. There was still much more to do.

First of all, there was the matter of registration, for which we had to line up and wait, even before starting on the paper work. Then there were the hostel rules with which everyone was required to be familiar. Our beds had to be made up with the sheets, pillows and blankets issued to us. And of course we had to unpack our belongings and organize everything we would need in our temporary quarters. It was 10:00 p.m. before all these things were done and we could get to bed.

So ended our first day in Australia. I hoped we would never experience another one like it.

Room 105

Chapter 3

Bonegilla Migrant Hostel was situated in the rolling hills of northern Victoria. It had once been an army camp. Its 40 or so buildings were typically Australian with their native hardwood walls and corrugated iron roofs. Most of these buildings were barracks, each shared by several families. Bonegilla had its own administrative block, general store and medical clinic. There were also a schoolhouse and chapel. The landscape was unlike anything I had experienced in Europe. There were no dark green pine-covered mountains around Bonegilla. All one saw were dry brown hills with only a sparse covering of spindly eucalypts.

Within the little settlement itself, however, there were several very large eucalypts—enormous white-trunked gum trees with giant branches. There was one of these magnificent specimens right next to our barracks. I first saw it the morning after we arrived. Its massive size dwarfed every building on the site. But what impressed me most of all was the fact that it was home to a variety of native birds. They chirped, chattered and screeched incessantly as they fluttered about in the attic of its upper branches some hundred feet above my head. And what colors! The pink breast and gray wing of the galah, the yellow crest of the white cockatoo, the vibrant purples, greens, blues and oranges of the lorikeet and his parrot cousins.

I had never expected to see such wonderful bird-life outside a zoo. Yet here it was in all its pristine profusion. It was with equal delight that I saw my first wild kangaroo; not in the remote outback but just a few hundred yards from the front door of our barracks.

After a few days, Marianne, the girls and I began to unwind and even enjoy hostel life. It was far more pleasant than we had expected. We were served three wholesome meals every day, for which we were charged nothing. We were not even required to wash our own dishes. While our children were being cared for in the kindergarten and child-minding facility, we were free to write letters to our families. We also wrote a brief note to Jack Lehman in Woolgoolga, telling him we had arrived.

In general, the place began to take on a kind of holiday atmosphere in which we found it easy to relax.

On February 24, 1969, we received a letter from Jack Lehman. He had responded to our note by return mail. Jack confirmed that our accommodations were still available on his ranch and that there would be work for me.

We were both elated. At last, it seemed, things were beginning to work out in our favor. Marianne and I began to look forward to our new life—in Woolgoolga.

****

"We're here, folks," said Jack Lehman, "this is Woolgoolga."

With puzzlement we all peered through the windshield of Jack's 1951 Ford V8 Custom sedan. All we could see was a large white Indian temple perched on the crest of the hill ahead; its walls, tower, and onion-shaped cupola topped with a silver-balled spire, dazzling in the bright morning sun.

"We've got a lot of Indians living around here," added Jack, "that's a Sikh temple up there. Woolgoolga township is just over this hill and down a bit." Jack turned off the highway and drove along a dusty road through the bush. One got the impression that the car, in which he collected us from Coffs Harbour Railway Station, was far too big for him. He seemed to be constantly stretching his neck to see over the dash-board.

When we reached the crest of the hill, we saw it; the place we'd just traveled 800 miles by train and car to reach—Woolgoolga. And even then, there wasn't much to see—a 19th Century two-story hotel decorated with iron lace, several clap-board shops with skinny verandah posts, and an assortment of drab, post-war fiber-board houses; many of them sitting on high wooden stumps above the floodwater level of Woolgoolga Creek, some of them sadly neglected, most of them tatty.

Since it was only 6:00 a.m., there was nobody about. The tiny barber shop was not yet open. Nor was the little turn-of-the-century drapery store next to it. Roy Atkins' butcher shop was not yet open for business. It was little more than a tin-roofed wooden shed that bore on its facade above the verandah, the rather pretentious name "The Meat Palace."

As we drove along Woolgoolga's sleepy little main street, I tried to imagine Marianne, with Claudia and Sandra, doing her shopping here. *It wouldn't be much like shopping in Paris*, I thought.

Jack drove on, past the camping park and up a steep hill.

"Look, Mummy, there's the sea!" said Claudia as we reached its summit. She'd seen lakes before, but she'd never actually seen the sea.

Jack had driven us onto a headland which overlooked the azure-blue waters of the South Pacific Ocean. "What do you think of that?" he asked, as he pulled on the hand-brake.

"Oh, Jack, it's breathtaking!" gasped Marianne as she climbed out of the car with the girls. We all stood there, our hair fluttering in the wind, overwhelmed by the beauty of the place. Golden surf-fringed beaches curved away to green headlands for miles on either hand—right to the horizon. Inland, a chain of mountains stretched north and south, most of them clad to the summit with banana plantations.

"I live over there," Jack said, pointing to a spot north-west of Woolgoolga, in the foothills of the mountains.

"Where is it?" asked Marianne, holding her hair back from her eyes. "Where's the ranch? I can't make it out, Jack."

"You can't see the actual ranch from here," he said, putting his arm around her shoulder and pointing to a tree-covered prominence, he added, "see that hill over there? That's where it is. That's Hacienda Santa Fe. I'll take you there now."

In barely five minutes we were there.

Jack's Hacienda Santa Fe ranch was a 120-acre beef cattle property. On it he had built, with his own hands, a huge house which, architecturally, would not have looked out of place in old Mexico. He had built it in the classic colonial Spanish style, with expansive walls; several of them with dark brown log rafters projecting outwards at ceiling level. Several others had graceful arches. Some walls were topped with decorative facades. The doors were typically Spanish; some made of heavy planks and others of carefully worked cedar with ringed iron latches. Extending out from the house itself were high walls which enclosed a number of courtyards. With its stone walls, its tall palm trees and its lake, the place was very impressive.

"You must be tired," Jack said. "Come inside and we'll have a cup of tea." He ushered us into his dining room, which, in keeping with the external features of the house, had a tiled floor, arched doorways and brown-stained rafters.

"Mary!" Jack called out to his sister, "We're home. Make us a cup of tea, will you? And bring in something for the children."

We sat down as Jack chatted on. Jack was a great talker. He was interested in everything and everybody—and he loved children. After a few minutes his sister, Mary, came in. She was a woman in her late 60s. With a scarf on her head and wearing an apron, she came in carrying a tray with tea for the adults, lemonade for the children, and a large plate of biscuits.

After half an hour or so of morning tea conversation, Marianne said, "Jack, do you think we could see our house now?"

"Sure," Jack answered, "we'll go across there right away. Of course, there's no furniture in it yet, but there's plenty in my garage out in back here. We'll soon carry that across."

We all followed Jack through the grass across the hill. The house was about 300 yards away. As we got closer we could see it was a small fiber-board structure with a low-gabled, corrugated iron roof. Jack opened the front door and we all stepped inside onto the bare wooden floor of a tiny kitchen. All it contained was a sink, a wood stove and an old refrigerator. It was barely a kitchen, it was really only a thoroughfare with four doors—one in each wall, the front one, the back one, and one to each of the bedrooms.

"Where's the bathroom?" asked Marianne.

"There isn't one," answered Jack, " but you can all use the one in the hacienda."

I could tell from Marianne's expression that she saw a problem here. The hacienda was 300 yards away. This could present some real difficulties at night or during one of Woolgoolga's heavy sub-tropical downpours—especially for the children.

Jack sensed her concern and hastily added, "Of course there's a bush outhouse you can use just over there. That's a bit closer."

As soon as we had brought our belongings from the car, Jack and I left Marianne in the house with the girls and went across to get the furniture. When we entered the garage I saw that it doubled as a workshop and storage area with tools, bags of cement, timber and various other things a handyman like Jack would need.

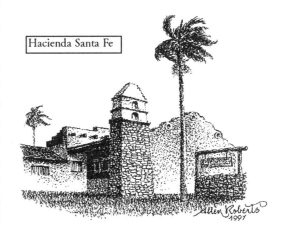

Hacienda Santa Fe

"We'll take the beds first, Marcus," Jack suggested, tugging at a heavy cast-iron bedstead that was lying under a pile of mattresses. "These beds are too heavy for one person," he said. "You take the front and I'll take the back."

We'd not gone half way across to the house when I felt a sharp painful sting on the upper part of my back. I dropped my end of the bedstead and reached over my shoulder to find out what had bitten me. Within the next second I was bitten twice more. I ripped off my shirt. Inside was a giant brown ant. It was at least three-quarters of an inch long. My back throbbed with intense pain.

As I shook my shirt to get rid of the thing, Jack said, "It's only a bull-ant, Marcus. You'll get used to them after a while."

I looked at Jack, my eyes watering.

I didn't believe him.

It took most of that afternoon to carry the furniture across to our house in the scorching heat. We made about 12 trips altogether—a total distance of over four miles. By six o'clock our little house was furnished, our belongings packed away, and our beds made.

Jack thoughtfully invited us across to his hacienda for dinner. We all showered in his bathroom, then, exhausted by the constant travel and work of the last two days, went home to bed. It was of no consequence to us that some of our mattresses were hard and lumpy and that there were no coverings on our floors, or curtains on our windows. We were just too exhausted to care.

But exhausted as we were, deep down, we all felt quietly excited that this would be the first night in our new Australian home.

Room 105

Chapter 4

We took the next week to settle in. Everything was new and exciting.

How thrilled the children were when Jack presented them with a pet goat—the first animal they'd ever owned.

Although for Marianne the house was small and the facilities little more than primitive—no bathroom, no hot running water and only an old black wood stove to cook on—she adapted quickly and without complaint.

The safety of our children, however, was a continuing concern to us because of the dangerous snakes, spiders, and, of course, bull-ants, which lurked in the tall grass around our house. However, we took the view that, if Aussie families who lived in the bush with their children could get by, then we could too.

During this first week I helped Jack do some fencing on his property. I'd never done such hard physical work and each night I'd come home with my hands blistered and my whole body stiff and aching. I was getting into shape, of course, for the physical work I suspected I would soon have to do to support my family.

I decided I would take up this matter of a full-time job with Jack.

"Don't worry about it," he said. "Take your time. There's no hurry. The Australian government will keep paying your unemployment allowance until you get work. And besides, you've got a house to live in, no rent to pay, and there's plenty of food for you to eat here on the ranch. So just relax."

"But Jack," I said, "I need to work."

"Well, you can go on helping me here on the ranch," he said. "I'll pay you for the work you do." So for the next few weeks I worked for Jack. I did a variety of odd jobs such as fencing, cementing, and assisting with his Hereford livestock.

I also planted a little vegetable garden next to our house. I could hardly believe the speed at which everything I planted grew in this sub-tropical climate.

Whereas it took three months from sowing to reaping, in the cool mild climate of Switzerland, here it took only half that time. So in six weeks, I was surprised to find I had bountiful crops of tomatoes, lettuce, beans, cucumbers, potatoes and pumpkins.

I was also surprised about something else. I found that the more gardening I did, the more I enjoyed it. I began to feel at one with this wonderful new world that was opening up to me—a world of plants that were alive and growing, vibrant and productive. I began to revel in the loveliness of the lush environment in which we now lived; its green fields, foothills and forests, its bird-filled valleys and mountains. Though I was here with my little family in a foreign country, I somehow felt that at last, I was home! My ancestors, for many generations before me, had been farmers. Perhaps the land was in my blood.

One day Jack said to me, "Marcus, there's a fellow who owns a banana plantation about two miles away—back of my property here. When I was talking to him last night, he said he might have some contract work for you. He's an Indian Sikh. How about it?"

I'd been told that plantation work was some of the hardest a man could do. By now I was beginning to understand what Jack meant when he had said, "You'll have to unsaddle the horse." As a former business executive, now living in rural Australia, I reckoned I'd unsaddled the old horse and was about ready to saddle up a new one.

"I'll give it a go," I said.

At 7:30 a.m. the following Monday, I found myself standing in Mr. Singh's banana plantation. My job there was to be 'trashing.' I had no idea what trashing was, so Mr. Singh, turbanned and bearded, his shirt and shorts grubby brown with indelible banana stain and his canvas gaiters turned down over his boots, treated me to a demonstration.

Taking a two-foot long, broad-bladed machete, he led me up onto the steep hillside where his banana trees, known as stools, grew in long rows, about six feet apart. Taking me into the shaded corridor between two of these rows, he took his machete and began slashing away the dead leaves which hung down below the green ones that grew from the top of the stool.

I stood there, amazed at the speed with which he reached up with his machete, and dexterously flicked off five or six of the dead brown leaves that hung there about two feet above his head. Both machete and hand were a blur as he moved rapid- ly and rhythmically around the stool in a kind of dance. With his dark, hairy arms and legs constantly mov- ing, he reminded me of a nimble cir- cus monkey. Without a pause, he went on to the next stool, then the next, trashing each with lightning speed.

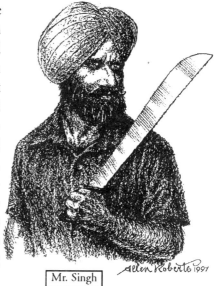

Mr. Singh

Then he handed me the machete.

I was highly embarrassed as he watched me grab each leaf with my left hand then slash at it—sometimes two or three times—with my machete. I was relieved when he went away and left me to build up my proficiency and speed. Try as I might, I just couldn't get the hang of it.

But I persevered.

Surely if my boss can do it, I can, I thought as I reached up and grabbed another leaf. Suddenly, a gigantic brown spider leaped out from under it and scurried down the stool barely a few inches from my face. I recoiled in horror from the repulsive creature with its fat body and enormous leg-span—almost as wide as a saucer.

My heart pounded as I stood there motionless, afraid to touch another leaf. Next time, would I put my hand on one of them? Or even worse, would another of the loathsome things spring out on to my face? The very thought sent a shiver down my spine.

It took me about 20 minutes to trash only 50 stools. It was very tiring work. By the time Mr. Singh came back, my arms and neck were beginning to really ache. Seeing that I was making such heavy weather of it, he took my machete from me and gave me yet another demonstration of his monkey dance. Once more he went off, leaving me to have some more practice.

By 4:30 p.m. it was knock-off time. Exhausted, I trudged down the hill to Mr. Singh's Land Rover so he could drive me home. It did not take me long to realize that I wouldn't be able to fulfill my contract of 3,000 stools in three days. It didn't take Mr. Singh long to figure that either.

It was a whole week before I finished trashing my 3,000-stool quota. By that time, both Mr. Singh and I felt that it would not be financially desirable to renew my trashing contract.

On Friday afternoon, I gingerly climbed down from Mr. Singh's Land Rover and walked with considerable difficulty to the door of our little cottage. I had the distinct impression that my newly saddled horse had thrown me—rather heavily.

That night I told Jack that I didn't think I was cut out for trashing and, for that reason, decided it might be time to call it quits. He didn't appear to be the least bit concerned.

"Don't worry about it, Marcus," he said cheerfully. "We'll get you another job. Tomorrow we'll go and see Clarrie Moller. He lives across in Woolgoolga township here. He's got a plantation about 10 miles north. He'll have a job for you."

"If it's trashing I'm not interested, Jack."

"Oh no—he'll have plenty of other jobs," he said.

Next morning we drove to the Moller's home in Woolgoolga. Jack and I stepped up onto the front verandah of their old, clapboard house.

"Anybody home?" Jack called out as he knocked on the front door.

A middle-aged woman appeared behind the screen door. She was short and plump with graying, curly hair. She stepped out onto the verandah.

"This is Marcus Luedi, a friend of mine from Switzerland," said Jack.

"Hullo," I said, reaching out to shake her hand.

Reluctantly, she let me take her hand.

"What had I done wrong?" I wondered. In Switzerland it was normal etiquette to shake a lady's hand when introduced to her. But on this occasion, I felt, that by doing so, I had made a bad impression—and on my potential boss's wife, too!

I was later to learn that in Australia the gentleman does not, on such an occasion, shake the lady's hand, and she does not proffer it.

At least that's the way it was in 1969. But things have changed a great deal since then.

"I wonder whether Marcus might get a job on your plantation," said Jack.

"Clarrie!" Mrs. Moller called out, "there's someone here to see you!"

In a few moments her husband emerged. He was fair-complexioned, tall, broad-shouldered, and muscular. When I was introduced to him he seemed far more friendly than his wife had been. He shook my hand firmly and, when Jack told him I needed work, stroked his stubbly chin and said, "As a matter of fact, I could use another fella on the plantation. Would y' like to start on Monday?"

"Yes, I would, Mr. Moller. Thank you." I said.

"We start every mornin' at 7:00. If y' come down to the Pacific Highway at 6:30 a.m. we'll pick y' up in the Land Rover."

On Monday morning, as soon as we arrived at the Moller plantation, I could see that it was a well-organized and productive outfit.

"Marcus," said Mr. Moller, "you follow me and I'll show y' what to do." We walked up a steep slope between the stools until we reached the summit of a 300-foot hill.

"I'm goin' to start cuttin' bunches now," he said, "and all you 'ave to do is carry 'em down that slope to the truck. Can y' see it below there?" he said, pointing down between the stools. I nodded.

"Are y' ready, Marcus?"

"Yes," I answered.

"Okay, just stand 'ere next to me."

I stood close by him.

Mr. Moller reached up to a large bunch on one of the stools (there is only one bunch on each stool). Then with two deft strokes of his machete, he cut two deep nicks into the top section of the stool from which the bunch hung. Then he reached up and bent the stool over with the bunch still attached, so that he could support it on his knee. With one more cut, the bunch was severed. He dropped the machete and with one heave, lifted the bananas onto my shoulder.

I grabbed the stalk to hold them in place. They were far heavier than I had expected. This bunch was around 70 pounds—about the weight of a seven-year-old child.

I began on my journey down the hill. It was difficult to keep my balance and I used my free hand to steady myself against the stools whenever I slid on the slippery, wet slope. Every step downwards made the bunch on my back jolt into my shoulder. When I reached the truck, my back was already tender and sore.

I unloaded my bunch, being careful not to bruise any of the fruit, then began my climb back up the hill. By the time I reached the spot where Mr. Moller had been, there were several more freshly-cut bunches on the ground waiting for me. So I picked up one of them and headed down the hill again.

This is how I spent most of the day.

The bunches I carried were, on average, about 70 pounds, but some were closer to 100 pounds. Occasionally I'd find myself having to carry a whopping big one that weighed about 110 or 120 pounds— the weight of a bag of cement.

Although the height of each ascent and the distance covered varied somewhat, I estimated that by the end of the day I had walked 10 miles; half of that carrying heavy loads and the other half involving a good deal of steep climbing. Depending on the steepness, the height of the terrain, and the location of the bunches, this job could involve a bunch carrier climbing 2,000-3,000 feet in a day—the altitude of a good-sized mountain.

By the end of the day, I was beginning to think that I'd rather be trashing.

When it was time to knock off, I was so tired and disheartened, I did not believe I could face another day of this. After Mr. Moller dropped me off on the highway near my home, I began to turn things over in my mind. I had just found out from him that I would be paid only $1.00 an hour for this work. "$1.00 an hour! What had my life come to?" I asked myself as I trudged disconsolately along the dirt track to our little fiberboard house. In Europe, as an executive, I could be earning $50.00 an hour. Although, admittedly, many things there were more expensive to buy, the plain truth was that, comparatively speaking, I was now a pauper.

Tears began to roll down my cheeks. At least I was glad that I was on the other side of the world where none of my friends could see me.

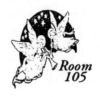
Room 105

Chapter 5

Somehow I kept working at Mr. Moller's banana plantation. I stayed there until July of that year; a period of four months.

I still do not know how, psychologically and physically, I did it. However, I do know that I was a proud man, something that Marianne had often said to me. She was right. My pride had to be dealt with, and for this to happen I had to be brought down—humbled. Now this was happening, although I didn't realize it while the process was going on. All I felt deep inside was a frustration and loneliness; a sense that I had failed my wife and family and that my life had amounted to nothing. Of course I blamed the circumstances at that time. But I now realize that it was far more than circumstances. It was God Who was using these circumstances to bring me to a place where I would understand my real need and turn to Him for help.

Curiously, God worked first through Marianne.

One afternoon when I was at work and she had put the girls down for their afternoon nap, Jack Lehman came in for a cup of tea.

"Jack," she asked, "do you have any books I could read—preferably in German?"

Jack knew Marianne was bored and needed something to stimulate her keen mind. He also knew that she had a genuine desire to learn more about God. So he gave her a book entitled *The Holy Theresia* by Tierstegen. It was about a remarkable woman—a sort of nun who lived in Spain some 500 years ago and had been persecuted because of her personal faith in Christ.

With her Roman Catholic background, Marianne was highly interested in the book. She asked Jack many questions, which he was more than willing to answer. He gave her more books, most of them about the Christian faith. Whilst he spent many hours discussing these things with her, Jack never tried to force her. As an old cattle rancher he knew that what was taken in, if it were to be properly digested, had to be double-chewed.

He also introduced her to some of his Christian friends who would gather together on Sundays to share their faith, either at the Hacienda, in the little chapel he'd built there, or at another ranch in Bonville, south of Coffs Harbour.

One day, Jack invited Marianne and me to come to one of the little Sunday church meetings he held at his ranch. Marianne accepted his invitation enthusiastically, since she saw it as an opportunity to learn more about God and the Bible. Also, she was lonely and craved the companionship of other women. I, on the other hand, accepted Jack's invitation with reluctance. But, because I was so beholden to Jack, I could hardly refuse. After all, he was far more than my landlord. He was my benefactor; the man who supplied our rent-free house and donated our supply of fresh beef, milk, eggs and , of course, all the bananas we could possibly eat.

So next Sunday saw us sitting with our children and some 20 or so other people in Jack's little Spanish chapel. I sat uneasily next to Marianne and the girls at the back of the sanctuary. It was the first time I had been in a Bible-preaching church for many years.

Jack and his friend, Alfred Bosshard, presided over the service. Jack led the hymn singing, which he accompanied—appropriately on his Spanish guitar. I was surprised by the volume and resonance of his deep bass-baritone voice. When a member of the group publicly prayed, I could tell that Marianne was following every word attentively. Alfred Bosshard presented a children's talk and his wife, Margrit, in a fine contralto voice, sang a gospel song. Again, Marianne listened with rapt attention.

Jack did the preaching that day. He stood behind his little wooden pulpit and, with his open Bible in one hand, preached with characteristic energy. Frequently, when he quoted or explained the

Scriptures, he would move away from his pulpit and drive his point home with large and often dramatic gestures.

No one fell asleep when Jack was preaching.

Clearly, he knew his Bible and loved to proclaim its gospel message; that Christ Jesus, the Son of God, died on a cross to pay for the sins of men, that He was buried and raised again, and that those who truly repented of their sins and believed on Him would be forgiven and have everlasting life.

Jack's message was not unfamiliar to me. I remembered hearing it in my father's church when I was a child over 20 years ago.

I glanced briefly at Marianne. She was hanging on every word. For her, Jack's gospel message was obviously fresh and new. She'd never heard anything like it in all her years as a Roman Catholic and was stirred by it.

But for me, Jack's preaching meant nothing. I felt I was an outsider and was glad when it was over.

Next Sunday, Jack invited us all to drive down with him and his sister to the Bosshard's ranch. The services were held there every alternate Sunday. Once more, I felt I could not decline his offer, especially since Marianne and the children were so eager to go.

Once more the gospel was preached.

And once more I felt alienated.

We continued to attend these Sunday meetings and soon began to establish friendships with those we met there. Although I disliked being in the services, I was willing to put up with them because the people who came were so friendly and kind to us. I was actually quite surprised to discover that they were even relaxed and fun-loving. I was especially pleased to see that Marianne had begun to form a firm friendship with Margrit Bosshard. Also our children loved being with the other children, and I had to admit that I also had begun to enjoy being with the men and their families; it was a welcome weekend break from the bullocking work I did on the banana plantation.

One Sunday, when the service was held at the Bosshard's ranch, we met a young Swiss man by the name of Jean-Pierre Reifler. He and his companion, Walter, had been traveling around Australia. Jean-Pierre was a wild young man and, as I was to learn later, an alcoholic. Although he had no interest in God, as a guest of the Bosshards, he found himself sitting in their meeting that day.

Something that was preached on that occasion pierced Jean-Pierre to the heart. After the service had concluded, as people talked in small groups, he stood apart from them, visibly troubled. Marianne had also been deeply touched by the message, and on seeing Jean-Pierre standing there alone, went across and engaged him in conversation. They talked together for some time about what had been preached that afternoon and in particular how, through Christ, a person could come into a personal relationship with God.

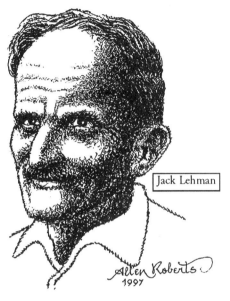

Jack Lehman

The following Sunday at Jack's place, Jean-Pierre was again one of those in the service. His friend was recuperating from an accident in the hospital, so Jean-Pierre had extended his stay with the Bosshards. Again Marianne discussed with him the questions raised by the preacher. They appeared to share a common interest in these matters and during the following weeks would often speak together.

I realized that Marianne was now yearning to become a genuine Christian believer. I also realized that she could not share her quest with me. Whenever I saw her discussing these things with Jean-Pierre, I felt uneasy. I was not jealous. But I was disturbingly aware that because my heart was so hardened against spiritual things, my wife could not even raise them with me and therefore found it necessary to discuss them with a man who was almost a total stranger.

As the weeks passed, my sense of alienation deepened.

One Sunday in May, Jack Lehman preached on how to be saved. He carefully explained from Scripture that one could be saved from a life of sin and become a child of God, only by believing on Christ and what he had done on the cross. He stressed that God's forgiveness for sins did not come as a result of good works on the sinner's part, but that salvation was a free gift from God.

When the service was over, Marianne and Jean-Pierre began once again to talk together. However, there was something different about the way they talked. They were more earnest than usual. I noticed that in Jean-Pierre's eyes, tears were welling up as he spoke. But his facial expression was not that of an unhappy man. On the contrary, he seemed unusually contented—almost joyful. Although I could not hear what they were saying, it was quite apparent from their animated conversation that he and Marianne were sharing something that delighted them both.

As they talked, Marianne caught Jack's eye. Then, quickly touching Jean-Pierre's arm to interrupt her conversation with him, she excused herself and went across to talk to Jack. She said something to Jack, who, when he heard it, smiled broadly, then embraced her warmly.

I looked back to Jean-Pierre. One of the men from the group had gone up to him and the two were now speaking together. Suddenly, the man shook Jean-Pierre's right hand, then, with a warm smile, squeezed it in a congratulatory, double-handed grasp.

"What was going on?" I wondered, as I walked across the room to pour myself a cup of tea. Before I had reached the table, Marianne came up to me. She clasped both my hands in hers and looked up earnestly into my face.

"Darling," she said with slow deliberation, "I've got something important to tell you."

"What is it?" I asked.

"I've just become a Christian," she said with the most serene smile, "a real one! This morning I believed on the Lord Jesus Christ! I've accepted Him as my personal Savior."

I looked down into her lovely, radiant face.

She waited for my response. I simply stood there—not knowing what to say or how to respond.

Marianne closed her eyes, then drawing close to me, laid her head against my chest. "Oh darling," she said, "at last I've found God. At last I know Him personally." She was close to tears as she added, "I'm so happy!"

I placed my arms around her and held her, silently, without emotion.

She looked up at me again. She searched my face for the response that did not come, then buried her head in my chest. "Oh Marcus, how I wish you could know the joy I feel in my heart right now!"

It soon became clear to everybody that not only Marianne but also Jean-Pierre had accepted Christ. For the next half hour there was a great deal of kissing, hugging and fervent hand-shaking.

As I watched all of these expressions of emotion, I couldn't help wondering whether this whole being saved experience was itself no more than some sort of emotional phenomenon. Would it last, or would it wear off after a while? I was skeptical and decided to adopt a wait-and-see stance.

I looked across at Marianne as she rejoiced in her new-found faith and shared it with her friends. Deep down I wanted to be part of it, but I couldn't bring myself to even try. In fact I felt cut off from her by all of this. I felt cheated.

In my mind I went back to the time before we were married. I loved this worldly girl so much then, I was prepared to give up every-thing to have her—including all the religious beliefs and life-style of my own dear family.

This whole thing had a bitter, ironic twist to it.

I, in choosing Marianne, had then abandoned the Christian faith. And Marianne, in choosing the Christian faith, was now, I felt, aban-doning me.

Room 105

Chapter 6

Now that Marianne and Jean-Pierre had accepted Christ, I realized that virtually everyone who attended these worship services had a personal relationship with God—everyone except me. As the weeks went by, I felt acutely, on every occasion when the little group met, that I was the odd man out.

But what really disturbed me was that I began to feel the same way when I was at home, because Marianne demonstrated, in everything she did, that she now belonged to a new and exciting world in which I, her husband, could have no part. From the day she accepted Christ, she began to change. Her bright personality did not change, but her character did. There was a greater depth to it; the old superficiality that characterized so much of our earlier lives began, in her case, to fall away. It was apparent in her relationships with the children, and with me, and in her day-to-day management of the household. It was even evident in her choice of clothing; the mini-skirt gave way to skirts with lower hemlines—still smart and attractive, without being provocative.

By the day she grew more caring, confident and content.

As her husband, I knew that what was happening to my wife was not some temporary change. It was certainly not the shallow, emotional experience I had skeptically surmised it might be. I strongly suspected in fact that what I was witnessing was an ongoing growth process; one of genuine and very possibly permanent change. This disturbed me. For Marianne a new dimension of life had opened up and I could not enter it and share it with her. My frustration was intense. I felt trapped.

During this period, Marianne developed a hunger to learn more about her newly acquired faith. To satisfy this hunger, Jack gave her a range of Christian reading matter, including a Bible, which she read every day when the girls were having their afternoon nap.

One evening when the children were in bed, Marianne and I sat at our kitchen table, as we usually did, and chatted together about the day's happenings over a cup of tea. I'd had a hard day and after we'd finished our second cup, I leaned back on my chair, legs stretched out and crossed, fingers laced behind my head and my eyes closed.

Marianne cleared the cups away and took them to the sink. As she rinsed them there, she asked, "Marcus, why don't you read the Bible?"

I opened my eyes and, looking straight ahead, said, "I used to read it every day when I was a child. In our home we were made to—at dinner every night."

"I've no desire to read it again," I said, closing my eyes once more.

"I found it boring," I added.

There was a pause as Marianne wiped her hands on the tea-towel and hung it on the stove rail. Then she came over and, standing behind my chair, put her hands on my shoulders, and gently kneading them, said quietly, "Darling, why don't you pray that the Lord will give you a desire to read the Bible?"

She continued to massage my shoulders, awaiting my answer.

I did not want to commit myself. Nor did I want to oppose her.

"I might do it," I said noncommittally.

****

The introductory hymn had been sung and Alfred Bosshard came forward to the pulpit.

"Would someone please open our service with prayer?" he asked, as his eyes roamed over the little congregation.

Instantly, Jean-Pierre was on his feet. Then with hands clasped firmly in front of his chest and eyes closed, he began to pray—fluently and confidently, as though he'd been praying publicly for years.

I was astonished. "How could Jean-Pierre have learned to pray like this in just a few short weeks?" I asked myself. In his voice and demeanor there was a sincerity and a conviction I would never have thought possible.

I could scarcely believe what I was seeing and hearing. It was like some bizarre dream.

When Jean-Pierre sat down, I knew that I had witnessed a kind of miracle. I now had no doubt in my mind that the power of God in Christ could—and would—change the heart of a man who trusted in Him.

Yet personally, I was conscious only of a bewildering belittlement and shame. Here was I, a 34-year-old man from a warm and supportive Christian family who had been faithfully taught about Christ from childhood and who, to this very day, had rejected Him. And yet here was Jean-Pierre, who'd had none of these advantages, now a new man in Christ. I also knew, to my shame, that because of the hardness of my proud heart, God had chosen to use this man, rather than me, to help bring my own wife to Christ!

I was shattered.

I sat in that little room oblivious to the people around me. For the first time in my life, I was alone with my God. I knew I was stranded there—with nowhere else to go.

In the quietness of my heart I simply said, "Jesus, I want to follow You. Save me."

I knew in that moment that I had trusted Christ.

I felt no great emotion and, throughout the rest of the service, gave no outward indication of what had happened.

As soon as the service was over, Marianne turned to me and took my hand. Then she kissed me and held me tight. She somehow knew what had happened.

As I held her in my arms, I said, "Darling, I've accepted Christ. I'm a Christian too now."

Still, there was no great emotion in my heart. I wondered why. I had often heard that when people trusted Christ they were deeply moved emotionally, almost ecstatically, to a level of transcendent joy.

I felt none of this. And whilst I knew I'd really been saved, it inwardly troubled me.

Why did I not experience the deep joy a true believer should know?

I felt as though there was still something I needed to do; not to be saved, for God by His wonderful grace had done that. Of this I was certain. But there was something, I knew not what, between God and myself; some kind of barrier that had to be removed.

I had no idea what it was. But I knew that it was somehow my responsibility, and that until I found it, and dealt with it, I would never know God's fullness of joy.

I was very soon to find out what it was.

Room 105

Chapter 7

In the days that followed my conversion, I became increasingly concerned by the fact that I was not experiencing the same joy that Marianne and Jean-Pierre so obviously had.

What was holding me back? What was this heaviness in my soul? I felt I was carrying a strange burden. I could not explain it. Nor could I get rid of it.

I decided to pray about it, so went off by myself into one of the sheds near the hacienda. "Lord," I prayed. "What's wrong with me? Why can I not know the freedom and the joy that should now be mine? Father, please help me!"

Immediately following my prayer, a most curious thing happened. I saw in my mind's eye a television set—not just any television set. I knew that it was the one I had rented in Zurich just before Marianne and I had left with our little family for Australia. The memory of this television set brought with it an aura of most unpleasant memories. These memories pricked my conscience and it seemed that the burden I'd been praying about actually increased. I tried to thrust the remembrance of this television set from my mind. But it would not leave.

I remembered, that when I'd rented this set, I had entered into a contract with the leasing firm, that I would pay a weekly rental for as long as I had the appliance in my home.

I remembered too that I had paid only one such amount, and, because the lessors had not sent me another bill, had not bothered to pay them another cent for the following three months.

But worst of all, I had sold this very expensive item, although it was not mine to sell, in the garage sale we held to dispose of all our belongings. In all, I had defrauded this television company for a large amount of money—well over a thousand dollars. And I had done it without a flicker of conscience.

But now my conscience was working overtime. I wished there were some way I could put the matter right.

I can't do anything about it now, I thought, in an effort to rationalize the situation. *It's all in the past and in any case, now that I'm a Christian, I have been forgiven for all the sins of my past life. I must put all of this behind me and get on with my new life.*

Somehow my attempts to justify my doing nothing to rectify the situation, did not make me feel any better.

If anything, I felt worse—and there was more to come.

Another matter then came to mind. It concerned my valuable Louis XIV antique furniture. It was dilapidated when I first saw it in a second hand dealer's shop in Paris. It consisted of six chairs, a large round table, and several other items, including two ornate gilt mirrors. I realized, when I bought it for a ridiculously low price, that I would be able to restore it and resell it for many times what I'd paid for it.

In my mind, I now saw all these items as they were in our Paris apartment—carefully restored and lovingly French-polished. But as I visualized them, I experienced none of the work satisfaction and pleasure I used to feel when I looked at them then—only a sense of shame and self-loathing because of what I'd done with them. Before I'd left Switzerland, en route for Australia, I'd signed a Federal Customs document stating that I would not sell any of my belongings for profit within five years of leaving the country. I had willfully disregarded this agreement, and, without paying any duty, had sold my antique furniture for an enormous profit.

As I emerged from the shed, where I'd been praying and remembering all these things, I resolved not to think about it again.

However, after another couple of weeks, my illegal dealings, in respect of both the television set and my antique furniture, crowded themselves into my mind once again. And once again, I wondered whether I ought not try to do something to put both matters right.

As before, I told myself it was not necessary because God had dealt with my past and forgiven all. As before, I experienced no joy or peace about any of it and my burden continued to weigh heavily upon me.

Another two weeks passed and the challenge of putting these things right assailed me yet again. It was as though I was being haunted by the ghostly visitations of a television set and a collection of Louis XIV furniture.

However, by this time I was becoming acutely aware of what was really happening. I knew it was God who was dealing with me. Here I was, praying to be released from my misery and anguish of soul and God was telling me how to do it. I had to make restitution for what I'd done. Of this there was no doubt. I had to repay those I'd defrauded.

A verse which I'd learned from the New Testament as a child sprang into my mind.

"*There is therefore now no condemnation to them that are in Christ Jesus who walk not after the flesh but after the spirit*" (Romans 8:1).

This Scripture made clear what was happening to me. I was a new creature, a new man in Christ Jesus in whom I had trusted as Savior and Lord. But I was now experiencing the condemnation and guilt of a man who was not walking after the Spirit (that is according to God's biblical principles) but after the flesh (the proud selfish motives of my earlier unsaved life).

Little wonder I was not experiencing the joy and freedom that was intended for me as a newborn child of God!

I resolved to put both these matters right at once.

I wrote first to the television rental company. I told them I had not only failed to pay the required rental, but that I had sold the set and pocketed the cash for it. I went on to explain that I had recently become a Christian and wanted to confess what I'd done and pay back all the money I'd illegally acquired.

Next, I wrote to the Federal Customs Bureau in Switzerland, explaining I had made a false declaration concerning the sale of my belongings. As I'd done in my earlier letter, I added that because I was now a Christian I needed to confess all this and make financial restitution for it.

I was aware, as I sealed each of these letters, that what I was doing would probably result in my being encumbered with a very large debt. However, I was determined to do it, regardless of the consequences. I told Marianne of my resolve and she agreed that I should go ahead, regardless of what it might cost us.

I drove to Woolgoolga Post Office and slipped both letters into the mail box there.

At the very instant they left my hand, a most remarkable thing happened. The terrible weight I had been carrying for so long suddenly lifted. At last, I was free! And most wonderful of all, a joy and peace of heart I had never known before flooded my soul.

I hurried home to share what had happened with Marianne. As soon as she saw me, she knew that God had wrought a profound change in my life. We both knew, that for the first time, we shared a faith that was at last positive and dynamic; a faith that would enable us to grow spiritually as one.

The next two weeks were the happiest of my married life. I was now able to share with my wife and my children the delight I derived daily from my study of the Bible and my personal relationship with Christ. My alienation from Marianne, Jean-Pierre and the others in the fellowship was gone completely. I now could see how God had used my loneliness and depression to bring me to genuine repentance, restitution—and joy.

I had a fervent desire to thank Him for what He had done through the whole process—not only privately in my times of prayer, but publicly. So I shared this latest development with the people who attended our Sunday afternoon services.

The reply to my letter about the television set came back with surprising rapidity—almost by return mail. The envelope contained no letter; only an invoice rendered for the outstanding rental and the cost of the television set. As I expected, the total amount I owed was well in excess of a $1,000. Fortunately I was able to pay it, and did so right away.

I wondered what kind of response my letter to the Swiss Customs people would bring.

I was aware that my false declaration and the illegal sale of my goods could easily result in my incurring a huge debt, along with fines and even prosecution. Now I could only prayerfully await their reply.

It did not come for some two months. On the day it finally arrived at Woolgoolga Post Office, Jack Lehman picked it up along with his mail.

"Here's your letter from Swiss Customs," he said, knowing exactly what I'd done to deserve it.

With some trepidation, I tore open the envelope and removed its contents—another single sheet, but this time not an invoice but a letter. It was typed on official Customs Department stationery, its letterhead in three languages; French, German and Italian. My eyes skipped cursorily down the page. Even at a glance, I could see that this was not the kind of letter one would normally expect from the bureaucrats of a government authority. There was no citing of laws I had broken or regulations I had infringed. Nor were there any amounts I was required to pay.

I began to read it carefully. It began with an acknowledgment of my letter, then went on to thank me for my honesty in divulging what I'd done. In view of the circumstances, the customs authority did not want to burden me with further proceedings and had decided to release me from all legal and financial obligations in respect of the matter.

The letter concluded by wishing me well and expressing the hope that I and my family would be happy in the country to which we had emigrated.

I was overjoyed, and shared this letter also with the fellowship at its next meeting.

Little did I realize that this sharing of my restitution experience would move others to respond in like fashion. This is precisely what happened to Jean-Pierre. Towards the end of that year, in November, two Swiss evangelists visited the fellowship on their way home from the mission-field in New Guinea. One of them was my Uncle Ernst who was keen to see me—especially now that I'd become a Christian. The other was Heinrich Müller. Immediately they had both been introduced to the congregation at the Bosshard's ranch, Jean-Pierre went to Heinrich and said, as he shook his hand, "Mr. Müller, I noticed that your dialect is like my own. You must be from the Zurich region. Am I right?"

"Yes, you are!" replied Heinrich enthusiastically. "I come from

Winterthur."

"Winterthur!" exclaimed Jean-Pierre, "Why, that's my home town!"

For the next few minutes the two gleefully exchanged information about the city of Winterthur, where they lived, where they had worked, and places they both knew.

There was a momentary lull in the conversation. Then Jean-Pierre, with eyebrows raised and narrowing eyes, looked at Heinrich and in a serious tone asked, "Do you know the Migros Supermarket in the suburb of Neuwiesen?"

"Yes, of course," replied Heinrich. "We often do our shopping there."

"When you return to Winterthur, would you mind going to that supermarket and contacting the manager there for me?"

"I'd be pleased to, Jean-Pierre," he answered. "Is there something you'd like me to get from the manager for you?"

"No," said Jean-Pierre, "There's nothing I need to get from him. But there is something I need to give him." After a pause, Jean-Pierre added, "It's some money, actually. You see, Brother, several years ago, when I was a teenager, I stole some items from that supermarket and now, as a Christian, I need to put the matter right."

"I used to make a practice," Jean-Pierre continued, "of stealing stationery from there and selling it to my classmates at school. One day, the manager caught me in the act and apprehended me. When he demanded to know my name, I gave him the name and the address of one of my school mates. He contacted the police and they went to the address I'd given. Of course, when the police asked to see the young lad whom I'd falsely named, it soon became obvious that he was not the culprit. In fact his parents supplied a watertight alibi for him. I, on the other hand, got off scot-free—or so I thought, until just recently!"

"I know," continued Jean-Pierre slowly, "that I must make restitution for what I did—in fact, I intend to restore to that manager twice the amount I stole. I also intend to write him a letter explaining that I need to do this now that I'm a Christian. And I'd like you to give him both the money and the letter when you return to Switzerland, if you will please."

Heinrich did exactly as he'd been requested, and in due course a letter from the supermarket manager arrived for Jean-Pierre. It was a warm and encouraging response. The manager thanked him for what he'd done, wished him all the best for his future, and added that if everybody would follow his example, we would have a much better society.

As a man with a former drinking problem, Jean-Pierre knew from the day of his conversion that God had brought him out from under the control of alcohol, that he might come under His control. The New Testament passage which describes this transfer of control is found, as Jean-Pierre well knew, in Paul's letter to the Ephesians (5:18).

"And be not drunk with wine, wherein is excess, but be ye filled with the Spirit."

Jean-Pierre, having believed on Christ and received Him, had already experienced the first part of this injunction. But now, through the process of restitution, he experienced (on receiving the manager's letter) the second part—being 'filled with the Spirit.' Jean-Pierre knew that being filled with the Spirit of God was all about life control. It was not how much gas was in the tank but who was in the driver's seat.

By voluntarily making good what he had stolen, Jean-Pierre was placing himself totally under the management of God. And by so doing, had experienced the Holy Spirit's infilling control. God was bringing to him a personal rehabilitation which would prove to be essential to the quite extraordinary ministry that God had for him.

It was several years before the spiritual import of what had happened to both Jean-Pierre and myself dawned upon me.

My subsequent study of the Bible revealed that the principle of restitution was a very important one that was set down in both the Old and New Testaments. Particularly telling was the account of Zaccheus, the tax collector, who, when he had a life-changing encounter with the Lord Jesus, paid back fourfold what he had stolen.

My later reading of church history also confirmed that God was pleased to bless and use those who made restitution for what they had stolen. Indeed it became increasingly apparent to me that on those occasions in history, when the Spirit of God moved through faithful preaching of the gospel to bring large-scale revival, soon after people were saved, they were often moved by the Holy Spirit to make restitution.

It seemed as though once a person had trusted Christ as Savior and Lord, and a vertical relationship with the Heavenly Father had been established, that through the means of restitution, God then enabled that person to establish a horizontal relationship with his fellow man. And this in turn opened up hitherto unrealized potential for witness and ministry. The history of the great Welsh revival of the 19th Century provided abundant evidence of this, as did other more recent revivals, such as the one which occurred early in the 20th Century under the ministry of W. P. Nicholson.

Nicholson, a working man's evangelist, preached powerfully to thousands of men who worked on the Irish docks. Night after night, huge numbers came forward to accept Christ, and once converted, began to return items they had stolen, sometimes over many years, from their employers. These items were so numerous that a large warehouse had to be built to contain them. The restitution continued and the warehouse was filled to capacity. As the revival went on, the stolen goods continued to be returned, until a second warehouse had to be built to contain them. When this too was packed to capacity, a notice was placed in the newspapers, asking that those who were planning to return more stolen goods, not do it because there was no place to store them.

Both Jean-Pierre and I sensed that through this process of restitution, God had graciously made us a small part of this great biblical tradition. We both sensed as well, that in some mysterious, wonderful way, God had used this means to release us spiritually, so each of us could minister to others in a manner and to an extent we could never have done before.

Room 105

Chapter 8

In September 1969, Jean-Pierre and I were given the opportunity to start our own commercial garden. Alfred Bosshard provided us with two acres of land on his ranch. Jean-Pierre and I invested in a trailer each and parked them both next to the Bosshard's dwelling so we could work our little parcel of land. Together, we fenced it, rotary-hoed it, and prepared its rich volcanic soil for a spring crop of tomatoes, cucumbers, and a range of other vegetables. Jean-Pierre, who had outstanding knowledge and practical ability in the field of mechanics and engineering, renovated and installed an old diesel engine and pump and soon our land was irrigated with water from the nearby river. Before Christmas our first consignment of vegetables was on its way to the Sydney markets.

By the middle of the following year, another opportunity was afforded us. An elderly gentleman who owned a banana plantation in the district, invited us to manage and work it for him. Jean-Pierre and I agreed to do this on a share-basis with the owner.

It went very well, and by the end of that year I had gained enough experience and capital to buy my own modest plantation. When I bought my plantation, Jean-Pierre went to work for the Coffs Harbour Mercedes dealer, where he was soon earning top money.

By the beginning of 1971, Marianne and I were well established on our own little property which was providing us with a reliable income.

As we approached February of 1971, Marianne and I suddenly realized that our compulsory two-year stay in Australia was now almost up. We were now free to return to Switzerland. However, we had no desire whatsoever to do so.

Whilst we would not describe ourselves as wealthy, we had everything we needed; a place to live, a modern Kingswood car to drive, and a regular income. Furthermore, our children had made the transition from Europe to Australia wonderfully well. They loved living in the country and attending their little school there. As a family, we were happy and we thanked God for what He had done for us. We firmly believed that He had brought us half way around the world to provide us with a satisfying life here in Australia and, even more wonderfully, had enabled us to experience what the Bible calls abundant life as Christians.

Now that we were established in our new environment and its language, I began to wonder whether it might be time to consider employment that might better utilize my former background and training in business. One day in April of that year, when browsing through *The Sydney Morning Herald*, I came across an advertisement that sparked my interest. It called for a Personnel Officer for the large bauxite mining firm of Nabalco, now operating in the northern part of Australia. I knew, from my business background in Europe, that this firm was Swiss-owned and a very solid, well-run enterprise.

After discussing it with Marianne, I decided there would be no harm in applying for the position to see what would happen.

Within 10 days, I received a reply from Nabalco, inviting me to fly down, at their expense, to Sydney for an interview. I decided to accept their invitation and telephoned them to say I would come. The next day, I was in Sydney.

At about 9:45 a.m. my taxi pulled up outside Goldfields House, the headquarters of Nabalco, in the bustling city of Sydney. As I stepped onto the sidewalk, the people thronged past me and the traffic whirled about noisily on the nearby intersection.

I felt uneasy. After two years in the relaxed country atmosphere of Coffs Harbour the whole scene was almost unnerving. Briefcase in hand, I entered the building and went up to the seventh floor where I approached the reception desk.

"My name is Marcus Luedi," I said, "I have an appointment with Mr. Zimmermann—at 10 a.m., I believe."

The receptionist, a young attractive blonde girl who wore a tight-fitting black outfit, ran her pen down a typewritten schedule and said, "Oh, yes...Mr. Luedi. Would you please take a seat, sir?"

As I sat down, briefcase across my knees, she picked up the internal phone and announced my arrival.

In a minute or so another young woman came in. She too was dressed in black and wore a very short mini-skirt.

"Mr. Luedi," she said, "Would you prefer coffee or tea?"

"Coffee, thank you," I answered.

As she turned and left the room, the unease I had felt, when I stepped out of my taxi, returned. Upon finishing my coffee, I was ushered into a very large executive suite. It was expensively furnished with a mahogany desk and several brown leather armchairs. It had a stunning view of the Sydney Harbour Bridge and the Opera House.

The manager, immaculately dressed, sun-tanned and athletic—a man in his 40s—came from behind his desk and greeted me. He spoke in Swiss.

"*Gruezi, Herr Luedi,*" he said with a firm handshake and a warm smile.

"Zimmermann," he added, pointing to himself—the Swiss method of introduction.

Then he introduced a tall, spectacled man who had been standing near the desk as, "*Herr Brunner.*"

Obviously the interview was to be conducted in my native language, which tended to put me at ease.

Mr. Zimmermann thanked me for coming to Sydney and we all sat down, not in the somewhat intimidating "boss behind the desk" setting, but in a cozy "armchair chat" arrangement. Mr. Zimmermann wasted no time in getting to the point.

"Mr. Luedi," he said, "We have thoroughly examined your application and we feel that you are the man we need for this important position of Personnel Officer."

He had my application in his hand and added as he perused it, "Your background in business administration and your training and experience as a quartermaster in the Swiss Army will have fitted you admirably for your work with us in handling personnel matters. Also, because we have a multi-lingual work-force on this project, the fact that you are fluent in several languages will be a great advantage too. Of course, we will give you 12 months training here in Sydney before you actually take up the position."

He laid my application down on the occasional table near his chair. Then, leaning back expansively, slipped both his thumbs in behind the upper edges of his waistcoat, "And, Mr. Luedi, there will be great future prospects, at managerial level, for the man who tackles this job effectively.

"As you can see here," he added, handing me a typed sheet of paper, "the salary is very attractive."

I took the sheet and saw that he was right. Then, after a pause to enable me to process the information, he said, "There will be significant fringe benefits too, Mr. Luedi. Every three months we fly our staff and their families to Darwin, the capital of the Northern Territory, for city shopping and so on. We would also fly you back to Switzerland free of charge every three years. Should your wife like to take a job, that could be arranged also."

I could tell that they had virtually decided already to employ me and that it was indeed an extraordinarily good position I was being offered. I was surprised and somewhat flattered at that moment. Yet somehow I felt none of the enthusiasm such an opportunity ought to have engendered.

"Mr. Luedi," Mr. Zimmermann went on, "our bauxite mining venture involves one of the largest foreign investments of this kind in Australia's history."

It was now time for me to ask some questions.

"Mr. Zimmermann," I inquired, "Exactly where will all this be taking place?"

He reached for a map and as he unfolded it said, "It's in Arnhem Land—'the top end,' as Australians call it, over 2,000 miles from here."

This appealed to my pioneering spirit as an adventure-loving globe-trotter. I knew that much of the remote tropical north was still largely unexplored. I knew too that this region was the natural habitat of the giant crocodile—a creature which I had long desired to see for myself.

"We are currently constructing a new town right here," he said, pointing to a spot on his map. "Mr. Brunner," he asked, "would you please show Mr. Luedi the town plan?"

I was astonished to see the streets, and buildings of a modern town, complete with school, parks and recreation facilities, including a swimming pool.

"It's called Nhulunbuy. That's an aboriginal name." He pointed to an allotment on the town plan and said, "This is where you and your family will live, and this..." he said, looking towards Mr. Brunner, who handed him an architect's plan, "is the actual house you'll be living in, if you take the job."

The plan showed a modern three-bedroom brick veneer dwelling.

"We'll make sure that you and your family are comfortable and well cared for. The house will be fully air conditioned and the block will be landscaped of course."

As I looked at the plan of this spacious, modern house, I couldn't help but compare it with the little cottage on Jack's property and the trailer in which we were now living.

"Well, Mr. Luedi, what do you think?"

What could I say? For any rational man, this had to be the vocational opportunity of a life-time. "It's great," I said, wondering as I said it why I wasn't inwardly thrilled by the whole thing. I tried not to show, in my voice or my manner, the weird apprehension I had begun to feel deep down inside.

"Splendid!" said Mr. Zimmermann as he rose from his chair and leaned over his desk to buzz for his secretary.

She came in at once, carrying a stenographer's notebook and pen. She was yet another of the highly attractive young ladies employed here at Nabalco Head Office. Like the others she was elegantly dressed. She wore a white silk blouse and an olive green mini-skirt.

Mr. Zimmermann took a small office chair and placed it in our little circle so she could take notes from him. I was momentarily distracted as she sat down and crossed her shapely legs.

"We'll frame up the terms of your contract right now," said Mr. Zimmermann, "and we'll have it all typed up and ready for you to take back home today. I'm sure you'd like to discuss it with your wife.

Is that acceptable to you?"

"Yes, that's fine," I responded.

"As soon as it's typed up, I'll sign it," he added, "and all you'll have to do, to make it a firm contract, is add your signature and mail it back to me in, say, a week from today. That would be...on Friday, June 12, okay?"

I nodded my agreement.

"Please make a note of that," he said to his secretary.

She noted it down and once more, to my embarrassment, crossed her mini-skirted legs. Within half an hour the interview was over and I was walking towards the elevator with a contract in my briefcase that I knew could open up for me a very lucrative career.

As I left Goldfields House and walked towards the Quay, what had been said during my interview surged through my mind. I was quite certain that, were I to accept the position I'd been offered, my family and I would be materially secure for the rest of our lives. Why was it, I wondered, as I watched for an approaching taxi, that I felt no excitement, no eager anticipation at the prospect.

Why was it that what I did feel, in the pit of my stomach, was a dull, ominous fear that this job would soon be mine!

****

"How did the interview go?" asked Marianne when she met me at the Coffs Harbour Airport.

"Very well," I said.

"Do you think you'll get the job?" she asked as we walked towards our car.

"They want me to take it," I replied. Then tapping my briefcase, added, "I've got the contract right here...all I have to do is sign it.

"Of course," I added quickly, "I wouldn't think of doing that until I'd talked it over with you—and prayed about it." Because of my strangely uncertain attitude towards the whole thing, I did not want to encourage Marianne too much, so I added, "We'd all have to go to the Northern Territory. As you know it's in the tropics. I think you might find the heat and humidity a problem, darling. They're much worse up there than here in Coffs Harbour."

That evening we discussed the matter more fully, but I did not tell Marianne that I had to return the contract within one week. We prayed about it together, asking the Lord to guide us in this major decision. However, neither of us sensed any leading from God. After a few days I could tell that Marianne was leaving the decision to me. So I tried each day to think and pray it through, while I worked.

However, whenever I did this, the whole Sydney scene, with its high-tech pressures and deadlines, rekindled once more the unease I had felt when I went there for my interview. Also, my potential career, as Nabalco's Personnel Officer, was somehow linked to my strong visual memory of that plush executive suite and that bevy of provocative, mini-skirted young office girls. What was also disturbing was that all of these images were in turn linked to the business world of Paris from which I'd fled just two years ago. But, most concerning of all, was that the vague fear I had first felt, when I knew I would probably get the job, returned each time I tried to pray about it.

As my contract deadline approached, I found I was no nearer to a decision.

In fact when Friday, June 12 came, I still had not signed the contract and tried, in fact, to thrust the whole thing out of my mind. I did not share my inner turmoil with Marianne.

Early on Wednesday morning of the following week, Marianne, unaware that the deadline had passed—or even that there had been a deadline—said, "Marcus, why haven't you signed and mailed that contract?"

"Darling, I don't really know what I should do. Somehow I just can't make a decision. I've been praying ever since I came back from Sydney," I added, "but it doesn't seem to have helped!"

"Marcus," she said sternly, "you can't expect Nabalco to wait forever. If you don't sign that contract right away, you'll miss out on the job."

Then, articulating each word slowly with obvious anger, she added, "It will be too late!"

Of course Marianne was right. But what she didn't realize was that it was probably already too late. The real problem was that I'd gotten caught in a kind of mental and emotional deadlock. I was incapable of making this decision. I went across to the little window of our trailer and stood there looking outside in silent, sullen frustration.

"I've heard that fasting sometimes helps," I said. "I've never done it before. But maybe this is the time to start. I'll begin at once. I won't even have breakfast. I'll fast for three days—and hopefully by the end of that time, God will make clear what I should do!"

So I fasted and prayed.

By Friday afternoon I had still not received any answer concerning my decision. I was hungry—and rather annoyed, as I took my Lutheran German Bible and went into one of our banana packing-sheds to have a private conversation with God. My conversation was almost a quarrel.

"I've now fasted and prayed for almost three days!" I said, "God, what am I to do?" In confusion and close to anger, I opened my Bible to find there some guidance on the matter. I turned to the book of Isaiah in the Old Testament, Chapter 58, I read the first section and, to my surprise, noticed a reference to fasting in verse three.

"Wherefore have we fasted, say they, and thou seest not? Wherefore have we afflicted our soul, and thou takest no knowledge?"

I was amazed to find in this passage that the children of Israel had experienced the very problem I'd been having—namely, fasting to know God's will and receiving no answer. I read on.

"Behold, ye fast for strife and debate, and to smite with the fist of wickedness: ye shall not fast as ye do this day to make your voice to be heard on high."

With shame I saw that my fasting was like theirs; arising from motives of anger, even a quarrelsome attitude towards God. I saw at once that I was really trying to badger God into telling me what I wanted to know—by fasting.

The following verse made it even clearer.

"Is it such a fast that I have chosen? A day for a man to afflict his soul? Is it to bow down his head as a bulrush, and to spread sackcloth and ashes under him? Wilt thou call this a fast, and an acceptable day to the Lord?"

I realized, having read this verse, that what I had been doing was not a true fast, but rather a farce. God was simply not going to have me use it as a lever to find out what I wanted to know.

Cursorily, I read the following verses of the chapter and saw that in spite of Israel's ungodly attitudes, God still had a glorious future for them, but only on His conditions. I was not really interested in these conditions and closed my Bible. All I knew, and needed to know at this point, was that my fasting, to know God's will for my big decision, had been totally ineffectual, and He had rebuked me for it.

I was still frustrated and angry, and felt as though my Heavenly Father had given me a stinging slap!

I left the shed and went straight to our trailer.

"Marianne," I said, "God didn't give me an answer!"

I quickly laid my Bible down on the table; open at the passage I'd just been reading. I pointed, without further comment to the first five verses of the chapter.

As Marianne sat down to read the passage, I opened the refrigerator door and began to search inside. "I'm hungry!" I mumbled.

Marianne continued to read as I began to butter some bread.

"I still don't know what I should do!" I said, shaking my head.

Marianne placed both hands in her lap and sat upright, still looking at the open Bible in front of her. "You might not know what to do, darling, but at least God spoke to you," she said, indicating with upturned hand the passage she'd just read.

"Yes," I responded, "that's true...but I still don't know whether to sign the contract or not!"

That night the fellowship had a men's dinner. Having broken my fast, I went to it. At this function I spoke to a friend of mine, a Methodist minister by the name of Dan Armstrong. I told him about my dilemma concerning the job I'd been offered.

"Tonight I must drive to Sydney," said Dan, "but before I leave I'll call in to your place and pray with you about it."

At 9:00 p.m. Dan, Marianne and I sat down to discuss the problem. After we'd talked it through and considered the Scriptures I'd read earlier, I leaned back, and with my eyes closed, shook my head and said disconsolately, "I still don't know what to do with that contract."

Marianne suddenly jumped up and went to the small mirrored buffet where we placed our incoming mail. "Goodness me!" she said, as she sorted through the envelopes there. "This morning a telegram came for you Marcus. Because I was distracted by a visitor, I forgot to tell you about it."

She found the telegram. "I'm sorry," she said, as she handed it to me.

I opened it. It was from Nabalco and simply said that since I had not signed and returned my contract in the agreed upon time, it had been canceled.

I read it to Marianne and Dan.

"There's your answer," said Dan.

In a sense he was right. The job was gone now. There was no decision to make.

But did this answer really come from God or was it only the result of my own tardy behavior in failing to sign that contract? I have since pondered it carefully and am now of the opinion that God used the circumstances of my Sydney interview to make me aware that I should not work for Nabalco. After two years in rural Coffs Harbour, God, through my Sydney visit, had plunged me back into the stressful environment of high-flying, upwardly mobile executives, mini-skirted secretaries, and wealth—all, I now realized, at a personal cost I could ill afford.

In this way I had been graphically shown that there was really no difference between the big business world of Europe and that of Australia—but I was different. I was now a changed person. And, as the Bible explained,

"if any man be in Christ, he is a new creature: old things are passed away; behold all things become new" (2 Corinthians 5:17).

Since coming to Australia, I had become a new creature and the old things of my past life had indeed passed away. They had not only lost their attraction for me, but the very thought that I might go back to them had become repugnant to me.

As a result, I had become not only psychologically incapable of making such a decision, but even physically was unable to take up a pen and sign that contract.

God had brought Marianne and me to the point where our old life had no more attraction to us. The challenge to each of us to forsake our earlier patterns of living had occurred in somewhat similar ways. Early in our marriage, Marianne, for family reasons, had given up the promise of a lucrative acting career in the film industry. And I, later, for reasons I did not understand at the time, had given up the promise of a lucrative business career in the mining industry. Whereas the decision for Marianne was a conscious one, for me it was largely a sub-conscious one.

Neither of us could have known that we both had to be free of these materialistic aspirations and involvements in the affluent world of entertainment and industry—in order to be fully available to God in the spiritual ministry for which He had been preparing us.

Room 105

Chapter 9

Jean-Pierre was a man of action. A man who, unlike myself, made quick decisions and put them rapidly into effect. Within 72 hours of his meeting Honi, a bright young Australian exchange student, just returned from Japan, Jean-Pierre had proposed marriage and been accepted. Within five months, they were married and making plans to exercise a full-time ministry in Western Australia. In May 1971, shortly after their honeymoon, Marianne and I visited them. As they discussed their plans with us, I wondered what the Lord had in mind for Marianne and me. There seemed little likelihood of our leaving Coffs Harbour to enter full-time ministry. Our family responsibilities and my plantation work would keep us here for several years more, I thought.

Jean-Pierre picked up a pile of books from the floor and set them on the table. They were texts on a variety of Christian subjects: Old Testament, New Testament, Theology, Worship and Preaching.

"When Honi and I decided to marry," he said, "I made arrangements to prepare myself for Christian ministry by doing some study and bought all these," he added, as he idly opened the top book. "But it didn't take me long to realize I'm not cut out for academic study," he said, closing the book again. "As you know, I'm a practical man. And that's what's needed in Aboriginal mission work. So we're trusting that the Lord will use us as we tackle it and, in the process, teach us all we need to know."

I browsed through the pile as I stood by the table. "You've spent a lot of money on these books," I said.

"That's true," said Jean-Pierre, "but I have no further use for them. Why don't you take them, Marcus?"

"What a wonderful idea!" Marianne chimed in, putting her arm around my shoulder. "Darling, why couldn't you study these books to prepare yourself for full-time ministry?"

"I'm not sure my English is good enough to handle that yet," I replied, as I turned the pages of a book on the Old Testament.

"But darling, you could at least start. You could study at your own pace. And I'm sure it could be done in your spare time. I'd do everything I could to help you!"

I had long known that it was the desire of Marianne's heart that one day we might serve God in some full-time capacity. I also knew that the Methodist Church of Australia had a home-study arrangement whereby one could prepare oneself to become an accredited local preacher, and then, with further work, could qualify as a church Pastor.

And so it was that when Jean-Pierre and Honi left for Western Australia, Marianne and I stayed in Coffs Harbour, where I began to study on a part-time basis for the ministry. Over the next 12 months I began to work towards my local preacher's qualification. Although I loved the subjects I was doing, I found coping with English at this academic level very difficult. In everything I read and wrote I needed a dictionary at my elbow. However, the discipline of the process, painstaking and laborious as it was, enabled me to improve my grasp of the language substantially.

By May of the following year, I had passed my exams and delivered my first sermon as a local preacher—on Mother's Day of 1972. I continued studying and preaching as I worked in the banana-growing industry over the next two years.

Towards the end of this period our third child was born. We called her Natasha. At the end of 1974 I was eligible to apply for a full-time position in the Methodist Home Missions Department. After being examined by a panel of Methodist ministers, I received an invitation to become a pastor of the Methodist Home Mission at Newtown in metropolitan Sydney. I was told, that were I to accept this position, I would be required to complete further studies to be formally commissioned as a Methodist Minister.

On December 15, 1974 Marianne and I felt that we should cut our ties with Coffs Harbour and commit ourselves to this ministry in Sydney—trusting God to help us faithfully to keep that commitment. So mid-February 1975 saw us all traveling in a heavily-loaded car towards Sydney.

The circuit steward and treasurer of the Church had thoughtfully arranged for us to have dinner with them and their wives as soon as we arrived. They told us that this meal would be ready for us at 6:00 p.m. in the house that would be our parsonage in Newtown.

We had left Coffs Harbour at about 9:00 a.m.—plenty of time for our journey and the necessary family *comfort stops*—or so we thought. But we hadn't taken Sydney's Friday afternoon traffic into account. Consequently, we were already late when we passed through the far northern suburb of Hornsby. And it was well after 6:30 p.m. when we saw the giant gray arch of the Harbour Bridge above the buildings of North Sydney.

We made two unsuccessful attempts to get into a lane that would take us across, and rather than make a third abortive attempt, I hailed a passing taxi and paid him to pilot us across the harbour to the city of Sydney and from there to Newtown.

It was 8:00 p.m. when we knocked on the front door of the parsonage. We were two hours late.

The door was opened by a brown-haired man in his early thirties.

"I'm Ken Smith, the treasurer," he said crisply, with a firm handshake. "Come inside. You must all be tired."

"Sorry we're so late," I said sheepishly. "But we got caught up on the other side of the Harbour Bridge."

"We're so sorry," apologized Marianne as she stood there with Natasha asleep in her arms and the other two girls by her side. "Dinner must be quite spoiled by now."

"Don't worry about it," Ken responded quickly. "It's only a salad. Leave your things in the car. We'll help you unpack later."

I could tell, from his direct, no-nonsense manner, that Ken was a sharp young man who said what he meant and meant what he said. I liked him already.

We all went inside and Ken introduced us to his wife, and then to the circuit steward and his wife. Our meal had not been long underway when Ken, who was sitting next to me, laid his fork down on his plate. Then, with commanding presence, he leaned towards me, his brown eyes holding me in their penetrating gaze.

"Marcus," he said, "there are two things you need to know as you take up the position of pastor in this church."

I stopped eating and gave him my full attention.

Then, with his index finger pointing directly at my nose and looking along it, as one might do over the barrel of a gun before pulling the trigger, said, "Newtown will either make you or break you."

His cryptic comment thudded into me like a bullet. I was reeling from it as I tried to respond. "Is that so?" I said, trying to mask the fear he had evoked. "And what's the second thing?" I asked huskily.

"Do you follow cricket?" he inquired in the same grave tone.

"Er, no...I'm afraid I don't," I said. "I really don't know anything about the game."

"You don't?" he exclaimed, as though my admission constituted some sort of criminal offense. "Then you'd better remedy that, Marcus! You'll never get anywhere here at Newtown unless you can talk cricket!"

In response to Ken's first point about Newtown's ability to make or break, I decided then and there that by the grace of God, I would join the make category. But as for his second point, about becoming a cricket fan, I resolved never to fall into that category—a resolution I have steadfastly kept to this very day.

We took the next week to settle in. The following Sunday I was inducted as pastor of the Newtown Parish. I was to be the second of two men appointed here. As I began to realize what a large and extraordinarily diverse parish it was, I was grateful that there would be two of us. It contained three inner-city churches.

The main church had operated in a gothic-style building for well over a hundred years. It was a spiritual home to large numbers of students from Sydney University. Originally built as a Wesleyan mission church, it had its own student hostels, food store and soup kitchen. As an inner-city Methodist church, Newtown was a hive of continuous activity, not only on Sundays, but throughout every day of the week—by itself more than a handful for any minister to manage.

The parish contained another church, known as Camdenville which served the high-density Sydney suburb of St. Peters. Although it was only a mile from the main Newtown church, it was markedly different in character. The min-

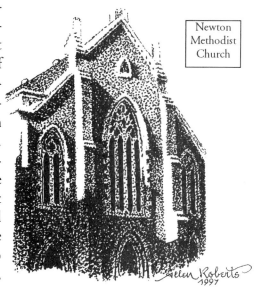

Newton Methodist Church

istry at Camdenville was essentially one of outreach. Its first purpose was to meet the needs of alcoholics, drug addicts, prostitutes and others who, for a variety of reasons, failed to cope with inner-city life and were dropouts. Its second purpose was evangelism and pastoral care for a wide range of ethnic groups, the largest of which was Greek, as evidenced by the signs on the shops in the main street. There were also Germans, Yugoslavs, Turks, Tongans and Fijians.

The third church was May Street Methodist in the suburb of Tempe. Its original building, erected in 1884 by the Primitive Methodists, had recently been replaced by a modern structure.

In addition to the heavy demands of regular preaching and teaching engagements, I was told that there would be an interminable succession of meetings, briefings and counseling sessions, many of which could not be properly planned in advance. I was also given to understand that most of the personal problems, which would flood in virtually every day, would already have reached crisis point and would therefore be very difficult, if not impossible, to handle effectively.

I must confess that I was taken aback when I found out that the superintendent minister, Reverend Peter Davis, would be away and therefore would not be available to help me through my first week of all this, which was to commence on the Monday following my induction. And what a daunting program it was!

I was required to spend five half-days (mainly mornings) at our Newtown Headquarters Office in the big gothic-style building.

During these time-slots I was confronted with a bewildering array of people problems such as criminal behavior, drunkenness, drug addiction, poverty, homelessness, sickness and family breakdown. To deal with these, it was necessary to work closely with the police, the law courts and the medical profession, as well as with social and welfare agencies. After my first day or two, I began to doubt whether I'd survive the week. How anyone could cope with such a program, week after week, was beyond me.

How pleased I was to see Peter when he returned on the following Monday. He and his wife Betty were an inspiration to both Marianne and myself. Peter's experience as a long-term missionary in Fiji, and his time as a minister in the inner-city, enabled him to ease us both into our complex and daunting roles. Without his sensitive and highly intelligent encouragement, we could never have settled in and coped as we did. We all felt that we were part of the Davis' extended family and I thanked God for them.

Outside mission hours, people in crisis began to come to our home—at any hour of the day or night. In this kind of ministry, it was often difficult, if not impossible, for Marianne and me to draw a line between our pastoral and our domestic lives; a fact that became dramatically obvious one afternoon in our second week at Newtown.

Room 105

Chapter 10

"Marcus, guess what happened today?" Marianne said as she greeted me at our front door. I had almost been run off my feet all day and was not exactly in a *guess what* mode.

"I can't imagine," I said as I kissed her on the cheek. "Tell me, darling."

"Just after lunch I went to answer the door-bell. It was a young girl with a baby in a basket. I could see she'd been crying and she said, 'I just can't cope...so I'm leaving my baby with you.' That's all she said—she didn't even give her name. Then she went off! And here was I, standing on our doorstep with this tiny baby—couldn't have been more than six months old—in a basket; no change of clothes, no food and no name!"

"Where's the baby now?" I asked. "Do you still have it here?"

"No, I don't. I phoned Peter's wife Betty, and she contacted the police. They came and took the poor little darling away. They said they'd arrange with the Welfare Department to look after it."

Marianne was visibly upset by the whole thing. I put my arms around her.

"Oh, Marcus," she said, on the verge of tears, "how could anyone—especially a mother—just walk off and leave a helpless little baby like that?"

We went together into our kitchen. I couldn't help thinking of our own little daughter, Natasha, around the same age. I gratefully thanked God that He had so directed and guided our lives that she was secure and safe with her mother in our little family.

Our home continued to be a haven for people who had nowhere else to go. Although most of them were grown men and women, they seemed to be just as helpless as that little baby left on our doorstep; no one willing or able to take care of them and the circumstances that controlled them driving them, into a cul-de-sac of utter helplessness.

This is how it was for a young woman called Judy, when she was brought to our doorstep at 2:00 a.m. by two burly police officers in 1975.

"Do you know this woman, Sir?" asked one of the policemen.

I was still barely awake as I looked at the freckle-faced red-haired young woman holding a two-year-old baby, obviously—from its red hair—her own.

"Yes, I do know her," I said. There was no mistaking her as she stood there in her skimpy little skirt. Her legs and arms were completely covered in grotesque tattoos—the pathetic cry for attention of one who had never been acknowledged or loved.

"She's come to our church occasionally," I said. "In fact I recently helped move all her belongings from St. Peters to Alexandria."

Then, addressing her directly, "Judy, what's the problem?"

She didn't answer. I could see she was too distressed and exhausted even to look at me, let alone reply.

"She's got another problem with her belongings, Pastor Luedi," the policeman said. "They were all thrown out into the street—with her and her baby—by the people she was staying with in Alexandria."

My heart went out to this gaunt little unmarried mother; little more than a child herself. Marianne and I took her and her baby into our home until the police were able to make arrangements to accommodate her elsewhere.

One of the most desperate and dangerous of cases, which landed on the doorstep of our home, was that of Lorraine. It was a hot summer afternoon in 1976 (our second year in Newtown) when I opened the door to a tall, voluptuous young blonde. Her sapphire blue eyes were wild with fear—one of them was almost swollen shut and her cheek bore a darkening bruise.

She glanced furtively over her shoulder. Then, her red lips

aquiver, pleaded, "Please let me in—I'm in terrible danger!"

Again she looked down the street as though being followed.

"Please let me come inside!" she implored again, her shoulders hunched and her feet moving nervously up and down.

I let her in and locked the door behind her. She was trembling as I guided her into my study.

"Marianne!" I called out, as I settled her into an armchair, "would you please make a cup of tea for a visitor? Make one for each of us, too, would you darling?"

The young woman was sitting tensely on the edge of the chair, her well-manicured hands nervously clenched, white-knuckled, in her lap.

I pulled my office chair across so that I could sit close by and directly in front of her. "What's your name?" I asked, as I gently took her hands in mine, in an effort to calm her.

She just sat there, tight-lipped and silent, then turned her head away as though afraid even to identify herself.

"I want to help you," I said as earnestly as I could "...and I promise not to tell anyone you're here."

I waited.

She looked at me briefly, then, with downcast eyes said "Lorraine."

"What's the problem, Lorraine?" Again I waited.

"I ran away from my boyfriend," she replied. "He beats me up all the time...and I just can't take it any more," she sobbed, her red-nailed hands to her mouth and her eyes closed tight, squeezing out the tears.

"You should leave him," I said as I handed her a box of tissues.

"I've tried—several times," she responded, dabbing an eye, "but he always finds me and beats me up."

"Lorraine," I asked, "have you reported this to the police?"

"Oh no," she gasped fearfully, "not the police! You mustn't tell the police, please!" She stood up and made to leave, as though she had already said too much. I went to her.

"It's all right," I said slowly, trying my best to reassure her as she stood there shaking, a wad of crumpled tissues held tight against her nose. "I won't tell the police, Lorraine."

She looked at me and said, "If you did, he'd kill me...this man is a powerful underworld figure."

The situation was at last clear. And I knew she was right. This young woman was in great danger and her very presence here in the parsonage had put us all at risk too.

When Marianne came in with the tea, I asked her to stay for a minute.

"Darling, this is Lorraine," I said. "There are two things we need to do for her urgently. Number one is that we must get her out of Sydney and into the country somewhere. Number two is, that she mustn't be recognized as we do it. She needs a total change of appearance," I said, as Marianne poured the tea.

"I'll attend to Lorraine's transport, if you'll attend to her transformation," I said.

Marianne looked at me over her teacup.

"Okay," she said with a knowing wink and a smile. In that moment, Marianne, the pastor's wife, suddenly became once more the actress who was relishing this opportunity to apply her little-used professional knowledge of stage make-up to such great advantage.

While Marianne slipped away to organize our fugitive's disguise, I phoned a friend of mine in the country and arranged a two-week stay there for Lorraine. I was just about to phone Sydney Airport to make a reservation for her, when Marianne returned with a make-up bag, a wig and a change of clothing.

Within an hour, Lorraine was no longer a fair-complexioned blonde. She was an olive-skinned brunette with dark eyebrows and black shoulder-length hair. She was totally unrecognizable as I drove her to the airport.

Within another hour, she was flying out of Sydney, leaving behind the brutalizing gangster and criminal world that had threatened to destroy her. Would these next two weeks enable her to break free permanently? Only God knew and only time would reveal it.

Without Marianne's strength and encouragement, I could never have carried on. No matter how frustrating and seemingly unresolvable the problems I addressed, she stood unflinchingly with me.

In no situation was this more clearly demonstrated than that involving Kathie.

Kathie was a very young grandmother—only 42 years of age. She lived with George in a house about 300 yards from our parsonage.

Kathie had two children, a 12-year-old son called Roy and a 22-year-old daughter called Germaine, who was no longer living with them.

The situation was sad. Both Kathie and George were alcoholics and their home was the scene of frequent drunken brawls. On a number of occasions these were so bad that I feared they might result in serious injury, so I phoned the police. Unfortunately, there was very little they could do. Kathie and George were but one of the many thousands of inner-city couples in whose relationship domestic violence was common.

Kathie, like many others in her situation, was welfare-dependent and saw Marianne and me as part of her support system. When she needed help, Kathie knew exactly where to go and what to do to get it. Furthermore, she attended our church regularly, every Sunday evening, when a meal was supplied. She knew all the religious vocabulary that would help her to ingratiate herself into our fellowship in order to exploit it. She could be described as a highly experienced and professionally skilled user.

One midwinter evening in 1976, around 9:00, Kathie's son, Roy, came to the parsonage. He was highly agitated.

"Pastor Luedi," he panted, "come quickly! Mum and George are having a terrible fight—there's blood all over the place!"

"Marianne!" I called out, "I'm going over to Kathie's. She and George are having a violent row."

Marianne came in drying her hands on her apron.

"Darling, please don't go!" she pleaded.

"I'll be all right," I said, as I put on my coat and kissed her.

"Do be careful," she said as she followed me to the door.

I crossed the busy road with Roy and headed quickly towards Kathie's place. As we approached the front door, I could hear—even over the noise of the heavy traffic—shouting, screaming and the shattering of glass. Every windowpane in the front of the house had been broken. The glass grated under our feet as we walked across the verandah. When I went into the entry hall, I saw blood on the floor and base boards.

Suddenly, there was a wall-vibrating thump and crash, as though someone had been hurled across the adjacent lounge room.

I went in.

Blood was spattered over the walls. Several items of furniture had been overturned or broken. The floor was littered with broken beer bottles.

George had Kathie in a corner. Her disheveled hair covered her eyes. Her mouth, chin and ripped blouse were covered with blood. George held her upper arm in a tight grip. He was about to stab her with a large kitchen knife which he brandished high above his head.

I lunged forward and gripped his wrist. I pulled him away from her, and held them apart until they began to calm down. I asked God to give me the right words to say as I grabbed some chairs and sat them down.

To my astonishment, they were both as quiet as lambs.

Although they were very drunk, I tried to get them to tell me what had triggered off this violent argument. Neither of them could, or would, tell me.

I then prayed with them and got them to promise not to revert to such behavior again. I told George, as forcefully as I could, that were the police to be notified about what he had done tonight, he would almost certainly be charged and end up with a hefty jail sentence.

I went on to assure him, that if it happened again, I would see it as my responsibility to report him so he could be put away. There was really nothing more I could do, so I left them to sort things out and tidy the place up.

As I stepped out onto the verandah, I saw someone standing there in the shadows.

It was Marianne! She had our large carving knife in her hand.

"Marianne," I said, "what are you doing here?"

"I decided to follow you," she replied, "and stood here ready to go inside if you needed me."

I put my arms around her and simply said, "Thank you, darling."

Silently, hand in hand, we crossed the road and headed towards our house. What a remarkable wife I had; so loyal and so brave!

I thanked God that He had given me such a precious partner.

Room 105

Chapter 11

The pastor of an inner-city church is frequently called upon to conduct funeral services. Because of the large populations of inner-city parishes, he is often called on to bury people he has never known, from families he has never met. This can sometimes lead to quite weird problems, particularly for a pastor who is under the tyranny of the urgent and constantly rushing from one unexpected commitment to the next.

One Monday morning, I received a phone message informing me that I would be required to conduct a funeral service the following Wednesday at 10:30 a.m. I was told that I'd be given the necessary details concerning it beforehand. Later that same morning, when I arrived at my office, my secretary told me that I had a funeral at 10:30 a.m. on Tuesday.

"On Tuesday?" I queried. "I thought it was to be held on Wednesday."

"No, it's definitely on Tuesday," she said, consulting the notes on her pad. I assumed that there must have been some mistake or misunderstanding about what I'd been told. So, I arranged, as was my usual practice, to go and discuss things with the deceased's family. I visited them that afternoon and, as usual, came away with all the information a pastor needs to lead a funeral service.

The following morning, Tuesday, I conducted the funeral as planned at 10:30.

On Wednesday morning, however, as I was busy preparing my Sunday sermon, I received a phone call at 10:30. It was from a very irate funeral director.

"Where are you?" he demanded angrily. "You should be here at the chapel for a funeral service right now!"

"But I took that funeral yesterday!" I said.

"Don't argue with me!" he snapped. "The chapel here is full of people and others are milling around outside. The service should be starting now. I'm sending a limousine around to pick you up!"

He slammed down his phone.

I'd barely finished dressing when the limousine arrived. Soon I was being driven towards the chapel, well in excess of respectable cortege speed. I was 15 minutes late as our destination came into view.

I realized, as we began to slow down, that I had none of the essential information needed to conduct the service.

I thought that the driver might know something about the deceased, so in near panic, I asked, "How did the lady die?"

"It's not a lady, it's a man," he said casually as he pulled into the curb.

"He was 44, I think," he said as I flung open the door and jumped out.

I was about to close the door when he leaned over and said, "On vacation somewhere." Then, tapping his chest, added, "heart attack."

I hurried into the foyer. Everyone was inside. The place was packed. Many were standing. And they were all waiting for me to conduct the service of a man whose name I didn't even know!

As I was edging my way through the crowd and heading towards the front, the funeral director suddenly appeared. He grabbed me by the arm and steered me down the aisle towards a lady who was seated in the front row with two children—no doubt the widow, I surmised.

Gravely, I shook her hand, as a sedate pastor who had everything under control, would do.

She introduced herself to me. This gave me the surname of the deceased. That was at least a start. All I needed now was his first name.

The funeral director motioned me towards the pulpit. As I

stepped up, he hastily slipped a card into my hand. I glanced down at it, as I took my place behind the pulpit and opened my Bible. On it was scribbled the dead man's name. With this minimum of information I began, and somehow completed, his funeral service.

It had been a close call.

One cannot help but wonder what would have happened if I had continued in my erroneous belief that I was burying a woman rather than a man. And, what a calamitous ecclesiastical blunder might I have made if the man's name had not been *written out* for me but was only *whispered* hastily in my ear? And, horror of horrors, what if it happened to be one of those gender-confusing names such as Gene...?

Out of this near-disaster came a wonderfully positive development. After her husband's interment, his widow spent some time talking to me. In the course of the conversation, I discovered that we had a mutual friend—a Christian lady whom we'd known in Coffs Harbour.

Within a few weeks, that lady brought her widowed friend to one of our Sunday evening services at Camdenville. That night, after I'd completed my message, I gave an opportunity to those who were not yet Christians, to accept Christ. The widow responded and that night became a believer.

****

"*Gute Nacht*," I said, as I shook hands with Jürgen, the tall heavily-built German with blonde hair. "*Auf Wiedersehn*," I added, as I shook hands with Peter, his Swiss friend.

This was the first time these two young men had been with us at the Camdenville Church and they'd both stayed on to chat after the evening service. The fact that I was able to converse with them in their native German, put them both at ease.

Because it was now past midnight, and I had a very heavy day coming up, I suggested that we all go home. Shortly after midnight, both Marianne and I were sound asleep.

Suddenly we were both awakened by the doorbell. It was Jürgen's friend, Peter.

He was breathing heavily. He'd been running.

"Marcus," he panted, the perspiration dripping down the sides of his face, "Come quickly!"

"What's the trouble, Peter?" I asked.

"It's Jürgen," he gasped. "He and his wife, Hika, are having an awful argument! Will you please come over and help sort it out?"

"Okay, we'll go in my car," I replied. "Give me a minute to get dressed."

Jürgen and Hika lived upstairs in a two-story tenement house. I followed Peter up the narrow stairs to their apartment. When we knocked, the door was opened by Jürgen. He seemed rather embarrassed to see me.

"Peter said you and Hika were having some trouble," I said.

"Oh, it's nothing," he responded. "...just a silly argument," he added, in an effort to make light of the whole thing.

"Could we come in for a little while?" I asked.

"Sure," he answered. Peter and I went in and sat down.

There was an awkward silence, then he said, "Hika's locked herself in the bedroom."

"Perhaps I can help," I said.

Jürgen went to the bedroom door and knocked on it with the back of his hand.

"Hika," he said, his head inclined towards the door, "will you come out please?"

There was silence.

"Hika," he pleaded, "Do come out. There's someone here who would like to speak with you."

Still silence.

"It's the Pastor of the Camdenville Church," he added.

"I told you," came the response in a Tongan accent, "I'm not talking to anyone—unless he's a Methodist minister!"

I knew that Methodism was the official Tongan religion. I understood Hika's insistence on talking to a member of the Methodist clergy, for they are highly respected in Tonga.

"Hika," I called out. "I'm a Methodist minister! My name is Marcus Luedi. Will you talk to me?"

There was silence again.

Then after 30 seconds or so, the bedroom door slowly opened.

And out came a slender little brown-complexioned lady, barefooted and wearing a brightly colored floral dress. I went to her and shook her hand.

"What's the problem, Hika?" I asked.

"My husband's a Nazi," she said, staring at him, her eyes smoldering. "And he wants to call our baby boy *Adolf*—after Adolf Hitler, because he was born on April 21, Hitler's birthday! And I won't have it!" she said folding her arms and setting her jaw. "My father says we should call our son David. And that's the name I want!"

"*David!*" exploded Jürgen, standing over his diminutive wife— menacing her with his huge bulk.

"*David* is a Jewish name! *My* father would kill me if I called my son *David!*"

He strode almost savagely across the room. Then he turned and drew himself up to his full 6 ft., 3 in. and, tilting his head back, intoned, "My father was a Nazi officer in the war. And I'm a Nazi too. What's more, I'm proud of it!"

He stood there almost regimentally, his shoulders squared and his heels together. I could not control the temptation to imagine him uniformed in jodhpurs, jackboots, and a brown shirt with a swastika arm-band.

He went across and opened the doors of a wooden cupboard. He reached in and took from one of its shelves a handful of German war medals. From another he grabbed a Nazi banner. He held them high above his head and, barely controlling his anger, said,

"Our child will be called *Adolf!*"

"He will not!" shouted his wife, her eyes blazing.

The atmosphere was almost electric.

I held up both my hands, and adopting the most conciliatory tone of which I was capable, asked, "Do you think we might find another name—one that might be acceptable to both of you? After all, there are thousands of other names, you know. Surely out of all of them you could find one you could agree upon."

Neither of them was impressed by my logic.

Then Peter, who had been sitting silently through the whole fiery exchange, suddenly gave his input. "Why not call him Rolf?"

To my utter amazement, this name was agreeable to them both.

I could see no reason why. However, it was just possible that Jürgen, knowing he'd never succeed in getting *Adolf,* settled for *Rolf*—a rhyming alternative.

In the final outcome, however, I suspected that Hika, although she didn't get *David,* may well have won this 'name game' on points, for when, in a special service at Camdenville Church, the child was dedicated and named, Hika scored heavily by having the whole ceremony performed, not in the German manner, but according to Tongan tradition. Not only did she obtain the services of a Tongan minister, dressed in national costume to perform the ceremony, but afterwards, she invited everyone in the Church to a lavish Tongan feast (known as a *Loo-Ha*) complete with tropical fruits and seven sucking piglets roasted in a hole dug, especially for that purpose, in our backyard.

One couldn't but suspect that Hika, plucky little Polynesian that she was, came as close to getting her own way as any woman in her predicament could ever have done.

Out of this extraordinary series of events came some spiritual outcomes which none of us could possibly have envisaged at the time. Both Jürgen and Hika joined our church and became special friends of our family.

Peter also joined our church and such was his commitment to Christ, that he soon became deeply involved in counseling. His caring heart and ability in this field were eventually to lead him into a full-time ministry overseas.

Room 105

Chapter 12

"Marcus, dinner's ready," said Marianne as she popped her head through the doorway of our living room.

"Thanks darling," I said as I stood up and led our guest, a tall dark young man in his late 20s, towards the dining room. Our three daughters were already seated—their faces bathed in the gently flickering glow of the tall candle that Marianne had placed in the center of the table.

"Colin," I said, "would you like to sit here?"

Colin took his seat rather awkwardly. There was uneasiness in his deep-set blue-green eyes as he sat there, bolt upright, hands on his knees.

Marianne untied her apron and laid it on the bench in the kitchen adjoining our dining room, then came in through the archway and sat down with us. We bowed our heads and I thanked God for His goodness, for the food set before us and, for Colin's presence in our home.

We tried to put Colin at ease as we started our meal. "We hope you'll like our first course," I said. "It's a veal dish, with potatoes, beans and mushrooms."

"A Swiss specialty," added Marianne, "it's called 'rösti.'"

Colin was still finding it difficult to relax. And no wonder. He was well outside his normal environment. I remembered what he had told me following our church service the previous Sunday night—the first time I'd met him. He'd been born, the child of an unmarried mother and had been woefully neglected in his infancy and boyhood. He'd spent almost all of his school years in institutions and, as a result, had entered the work force poorly educated and with little employment potential. His poor self-esteem and low level of confidence were observable in his hesitant speech.

Although Colin genuinely desired work and repeatedly sought it as a handyman in the building industry, he could rarely hold down a job for more than a few weeks. Consequently, for most of his working life, he had been supported financially by Social Security. With others, like himself, his accommodations had been a succession of derelict houses in the inner-city.

At 28 years of age, Colin was already locked into a pattern of alcohol and tobacco addiction which would, almost certainly, kill him if he were not fatally injured beforehand in one of his numerous street fights. He was a self-confessed dropout; a loner who bore a weighty grudge against the world that had treated him so cruelly.

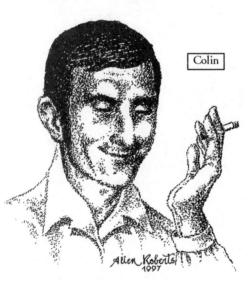

Colin

There were visible telltale signs of his sad background as he sat there silently sharing his meal with us. His unpressed checked shirt, his torn trousers, his missing front tooth (punched out in some drunken brawl) all bore mute testimony to his tragic plight.

Yet in spite of all this, there was something about Colin that set him apart from so many others in his situation. I had sensed it when I'd first met him and invited him to our home. I longed to help him.

My opportunity to do so was about to open up in a manner I had not expected.

He suddenly stopped eating and just sat there, motionless for several seconds, holding his knife and fork loosely, his forearms resting on the table on each side of the plate. He looked straight at me, his dark eyebrows raised in puzzlement.

"Marcus," he said, "I can't get over it!"

"Can't get over what?" I asked.

He shook his head in bafflement. Then, groping for the right words, said, "I just can't...I just can't get over the fact that...everything here," he waved his fork to indicate everything he could see, "...your family, your home, is all so...so harmonious!"

His candid comment took me by surprise. I didn't know how to respond. Then, before either Marianne or I could even begin to do so, Colin added, "I've never in my whole life been with a family, a real family, that is. All of this," he said, waving his knife again, "is a completely new experience for me."

"You see," he explained, "I've spent nearly all my life in institutions: places where nobody really cared for anybody else; where nobody showed love."

I knew that what this sad young man was saying was no idle comment. Nor was it said to impress or invoke pity. Here was the heartfelt cry of a man who had never personally known love but longed to know it now. It was a desperate cry for help.

This was my opportunity. So I seized on it at once.

"Colin," I asked, "do you realize that Jesus loves you?"

"Loves me?" he responded in disbelief. "No one has ever loved *me*."

"Jesus did," I said. "He loved you so much, that He gave His life for you." I opened my Bible and showed him the oft-quoted Scripture, John 3:16:

"For God so loved the world that he gave his only begotten Son that whosoever believeth in him should not perish but have everlasting life."

I got him to read the passage for himself. Then I explained that the only way to know and truly experience this great love of God was to turn from one's sin, in sincere repentance, and accept by faith the free gift of salvation available only in Christ, who took the punishment for our sins on the cross. I also told him that, although the Lord Jesus Christ had been crucified, dead and buried, God had raised Him from the dead and that those who accepted Him as Savior and Lord would receive the same eternal life.

Colin listened intently as I showed him the New Testament passages which revealed these wonderful truths.

When I showed him from Ephesians 2:8,9 that salvation could not be earned by good works but was given freely by a gracious God, he looked hard at the passage and then in genuine wonderment asked,

"Is it as easy as that?"

"Yes it is," I replied. "When I became a Christian, I simply took God at His word and believed on Christ as my Savior and my Lord."

"And that was all?" asked Colin.

"That was all," I replied.

I waited for a few more moments so that he could absorb this simple, yet profound reality. Then quietly I asked,

"Colin, would *you* like to trust in Christ?"

He looked me straight in the eye and said resolutely,

"Yes, I would."

"You can do that right now," I said.

"How?" he asked.

"You call on Him; ask Him to save you and He'll do it. The Bible says, *'whosoever shall call on the name of the Lord shall be saved'* " (Acts 2:21).

I was sure that Colin genuinely desired to trust Christ but just didn't know how to go about it. So I told him that if he'd like me to, I'd be happy to lead him through a straightforward prayer in which he could ask God to save him.

He readily agreed to my suggestion, then after I had briefly explained what it might involve, led him phrase by phrase through a brief scriptural salvation prayer:

>> "Before God, I confess that I am a sinner" (Romans 3:23).

>> "I now repent of my sin and come to the Lord Jesus Christ" (Acts 3:19).

>> "I accept Jesus Christ as my personal Savior" (John 1:12).

>> "I thank the Lord for dying for me and bearing away my sin" (Romans 5:8).

>> "I believe that Jesus rose from the dead and I will confess Him before men as my Lord" (Romans 10:9).

>> "I desire from this day on to live according to the principles

of God's Word that I might be pleasing to Him and fruitful in my new life" (Colossians 1:10).

>> "I thank You Lord for giving Your only begotten Son, the Lord Jesus Christ, to die for me" (John 3:16).

>> "In the name of the Lord Jesus Christ, I thank You that because He shed His precious blood for me, I am now saved" (1 Peter 1:9).

As soon as he had finished praying, Colin opened his eyes.

"At last I know somebody really loves me," he said.

When he came to our home that night, Colin knew that he was accepted into our family. We rejoiced over that.

But far more wonderful was the fact that when Colin left our home, he knew that, in Christ, he had been accepted into the family of God.

And the angels of Heaven rejoiced over that!

I felt it was important that Colin's decision to trust Christ be followed up as soon as possible. So I suggested that he begin each day by reading from the Gospel of John. I also made a special arrangement to have him come to see me regularly once a week.

On the following Tuesday, at 7:30 p.m., he arrived, Bible in hand, at our parsonage.

"How's your reading of John going?" I asked, as we sat down in my study.

"Great," he answered. "I've read the lot."

"You've read *all* of the book of John?" I asked, wondering if I'd understood him correctly. I knew Colin was a slow reader and was amazed at his perseverance.

With enthusiasm, he began to tell me about the things he'd learned and, as I discussed them with him, I realized that he'd not only read and remembered what he'd read, but had really understood it. Indeed, I was astonished by the depth of his understanding.

It seemed to me that the scriptural promise of Romans 10:17 was being evidenced here in this eager young convert's first encounter with God and His Word: "*...faith cometh by hearing and hearing by the word of God.*"

Colin then hit me with a barrage of questions. Many of them

concerned the teachings of Christ and how a believer ought to put them into practice. He posed questions as well about the nature of religion.

I pointed out that the biblically Christian faith was not actually a religion at all but a relationship. When he asked me to explain how the church fitted into all this, I told him that the true church was simply a group of believers, each of whom, like himself, had entered into a relationship on a personal level when they accepted Christ and that they worked together as a body to preach, to teach, and to encourage one another.

It was apparent to me that God had made him remarkably open to spiritual things. It was also apparent that what Colin had received that week, he wanted to share with others. He was no closet Christian. In the course of the past week, he had shared how he'd accepted Christ with his fellow lodgers, with his hotel mates and even with the young men in his street gang.

I could hardly believe that this young man, who formerly had been so morose, hesitant and self-conscious, was now so animated and excited about what God was doing in his life. He was quite lost in the wonder of it all, and, as he talked on, took a packet of cigarettes from the breast-pocket of his shirt. He removed one of them and lit it. So absorbed was he in our conversation, that he seemed unaware that he'd even done it.

He continued to smoke as we talked. It was not long before my study was filled with smoke—a situation to which Colin was totally oblivious—even when I stood up and opened the window.

At about 9:30 p.m. I prayed with Colin and made arrangements to see him again at the same time the following week. I saw him to the front door, shook his hand and waved to him as he closed the front gate. He waved back cheerily.

"Good night, Marcus," he said, "and thanks for everything."

I watched him as he strode off briskly into the night. I fancied I could see a spring in his step. Although it was a cold night, I did not close the door. After those couple of hours in my study with Colin, I felt the need to fill my lungs with some smoke-free air.

As I went inside and walked back towards my study, I thanked the Lord for having wrought such an astonishing change in Colin's life. I prayed that He would continue to bless and use him. I asked that through the Spirit's power, Colin's heavy addiction to alcohol and tobacco would be broken. I prayed too, that I might be able to encourage Colin not to call on his own strength to deal with these problems but to call on the Lord for His power to do it.

I'd gone back to my study and was tidying up my desk, when Marianne appeared in the doorway. "Marcus," she said, frowning and waving her hand in front of her face, "your study is reeking with cigarette smoke—it's through the whole house!"

"I'm sorry, darling," I said. "But Colin just couldn't help himself."

"Didn't he ask your permission to smoke in here?"

"No, he didn't," I replied.

"Then you ought to have stopped him," she said. "It's bad for the children and the parsonage is going to smell of smoke for days. As cold as it is tonight, I'll have to open every window in the house to air the place!"

For the next few minutes, I could hear her unlatching and opening windows and spraying each room with deodorant. Finally, she returned to my study and without a word sprayed everything in it—including me.

My wife, conscientious housekeeper that she was, was understandably annoyed. As she sprayed the curtains, I stood up and put my arm around her.

"Marianne, Colin's been a believer for only one week and he's going so well in his Christian life. I'm certain that the Lord will deal with his smoking and drinking—when the time is right."

I gave her a squeeze. "Colin's a special case, darling. Let's have patience, shall we?"

She snapped the lid on to the deodorant can. Then she turned around and kissed me pertly on the chin. "Okay," she said, "I guess I'll have enough patience to wait for Colin to quit smoking and stop polluting our home."

Then, patting my cheek, she added with a wry smile, "After all, I waited for three years for *you* to do it, darling."

The following Tuesday, as arranged, Colin was back again, but this time with a friend. "Hi, Marcus," he said when I opened the front door. "Do you mind if Steve comes in too?"

"Not at all," I replied.

Steve was a handsome young fellow, bright-eyed, broad-shoul-dered and muscular. He wore a white open-necked shirt and blue jeans. I estimated that he was about 25 years old.

As I invited them both into my study, I noticed that once again, the breast-pocket of Colin's shirt betrayed the cigarette-box bulge. *Oh my, we're in for another smoky evening,* I thought.

Although Steve had not yet accepted Christ, his interest had been so stirred by Colin's testimony, that he began almost at once to ply me with questions.

I handed him a Bible, so he could see for himself the scriptural basis of the answers I gave him. Within a few minutes, we were engaged in a three-way conversation-Bible study.

Once again, Colin became completely absorbed in the exercise and removed the packet of cigarettes from his pocket. Then, while I went on to comment on a Bible verse we had been examining, he opened the lid and offered Steve a cigarette.

Steve looked at me to gauge my reaction. I simply finished mak-ing my comment and waited to see what would happen.

Steve took a cigarette from the packet then looked back at Colin, who casually took out a cigarette for himself and let it dangle from his lips, as he rummaged for his matches. "You know, Colin," said Steve, "as a Christian you shouldn't smoke!"

There was a pause.

Colin struck a match and held it out to light Steve's cigarette. Then he lit his own, shook the match to extinguish it and slipped it back into the match box. Then leaning back and exhaling, a note of provocation in his voice, he asked, "Why, what's wrong with smok-ing?"

Steve made no reply.

So Colin turned to me. "Marcus," he asked, "what do you think of smoking?"

"I smoked for 10 years," I answered. "And I tried many times to give it up—without success. I was addicted, you see. It was virtually impossible for me to stop. But when I became a believer, I read the Scripture in 1 Corinthians 6:19, 20. This Scripture says to Christians: '...*know ye not that your body is the temple of the Holy Ghost which is in you, which ye have of God, and ye are not your own? For ye are bought with a price: therefore glorify God in your body, and in your spirit, which are God's.'*

"It was then that I realized my body was actually the dwelling place of God's Holy Spirit and, as such, should be kept pure and clean. I knew that nicotine would pollute, and, ultimately, might even destroy my body which really belonged to God now I was saved.

"Since I knew I couldn't stop smoking in my own strength, I handed the whole thing over to the Lord. I asked Him to take away the craving and break the habit permanently."

Colin was watching me intently. So was Steve.

"You see," I went on, "I was in bondage to cigarettes. And until that bondage was broken, I knew I could never experience the freedom that was to be mine in Christ. As the New Testament teaches,

'If the Son shall make you free, you shall be free indeed' (John 8:36).

"From the day I handed my addiction over to Christ and asked Him to release me from it, my craving for cigarettes was gone. I have never smoked or wanted to smoke from that day to this."

Once more, the two ensuing hours of discussion and Bible study were just as exciting and profitable as they had been on the previous Tuesday.

Once more, my study and the house were filled with the stench of cigarette smoke. As soon as our visitors had gone, I opened the windows and Marianne sprayed. We both prayed for an even larger measure of patience.

The following Tuesday evening, only Colin came to the parsonage. How relieved and delighted I was to note that his breast-pocket was empty. He could barely contain his excitement as he came into my study.

"Marcus," he said, "I'm free too! I threw all my cigarettes away! And I asked the Lord to take away my craving—and He did it!"

"Good on you, mate," I said, giving him a warm hug. "I must tell Marianne!" I went to the study door.

"Marianne," I called excitedly. "Will you come in here for a moment? Colin's got something to tell you!"

As soon as she came in, Colin said, "Marianne, I've given up smoking!"

"Oh, Colin," she said, throwing her arms around him, "that's wonderful!"

Marianne knew what a personal achievement this was for Colin because, like me, she too had been a smoker before becoming a Christian. She also knew that the three of us, who stood together in my study that night, had all been delivered from the habit by the power of God.

She stood back for a moment, her hands on Colin's shoulders, then hugged him again. "Praise God!" she said—and I knew she meant it.

"You know," said Colin, "I didn't even think that smoking wasn't right for me as a Christian—until the subject came up last Tuesday night, that is. And it was Steve who brought it up—do you remember Marcus?"

"I remember," I replied.

"Do you know, Marcus," he went on, "if *you'd* raised it and told me not to smoke I'd have gotten really angry—you know what a bad-tempered guy I am—I might even have punched you in the nose!"

Room 105

Chapter 13

Within the next few weeks, Steve also accepted Christ and shortly afterwards, he too, gave up smoking. It wasn't long before both he and Colin gave up drinking as well. There were also marked changes in their manners and general behavior. The former crudeness of their language and their habitual swearing disappeared. The grace and power of God in their lives was undeniably apparent to everyone who knew them and their influence touched many others, both in our church and beyond it.

But for Colin, one of the most remarkable pieces of divine rehabilitation was yet to be done. As a vagrant and a dropout, Colin had never, in the 10 years of his working life, bothered to file a tax return. But from his diligent study of the Bible, he began to see, that in order to live a godly life in Christ Jesus, there were certain responsibilities that had to be fulfilled.

Because he was serious about bringing his Christian life into conformity with Bible principles, he resolved to attend to the taxation matter at once.

As a first step, he went to the Taxation Department and told them what he'd done—or rather failed to do. He also told them that now he'd become a Christian, he was determined to put the matter right. The officials were surprised to hear this confession and, to begin with, didn't really know how to handle such an unusual situation.

But Colin was adamant. His misdemeanor had to be dealt with.

The problem was that he had no records of the 20 or so jobs he'd had over the past decade. Nor did he remember the times of his employment or the amounts he'd been paid over the period. However, he did recall the names of his employers. This enabled the Taxation Department to track down most of the required information in their computer records. They eventually got the rest from correspondence and phone calls.

The entire process took nearly six months of tedious work, the vast majority of it at Taxation Department expense.

Finally, the day arrived when everything was available for Colin to file his returns. They handed him 20 blank forms, then, since he'd never completed any before, sat him down at a desk and helped him fill them out.

Colin was informed that the Taxation Department would be back in touch with him in about a month. They also informed him that his failure to submit returns was a serious breach of law and, as such, a punishable offense.

On the day he received word from the Taxation Department, he called in to the Church office where I was working. In his hand was a long brown official envelope. He'd already opened it.

"Have a look at this, Marcus," he said handing it to me.

Inside was a check for $450—a refund made payable to him.

"Marcus!" he chortled, "can you believe it? *They've* actually paid *me!* This is the largest amount of money I've ever had!"

"How are you going to spend it?" I asked.

"I've already thought about that," he replied. "In about two weeks it will be Mother's Day. I haven't seen my mother for a long time. She's living somewhere in Melbourne. I'm going to use this money to buy her a present. I want to show her that I love her. I could never find it in my heart to love her before. But now I'm a Christian, I can. I reckon I can find out where she lives and when I do, I'm going to use the rest of this money to travel down to Melbourne and see her."

In approximately two weeks, Colin left for Melbourne, just as he said he would, and visited his mother there. He gave her the first Mother's Day present she'd ever received. Then he told her he loved her. He explained how he'd become a Christian, and that God had taken away all the hurt, resentment, and bitterness he'd felt towards her. He asked for her forgiveness, then shared the gospel with her. Colin stayed with his mother for a week, then returned to Sydney.

He'd only been back a few weeks when he suddenly turned up at the parsonage. He was in a distraught state.

"Colin, what's the problem?" I asked.

He made no reply.

I took him by the arm and led him down the passageway towards my study. On the way, we passed the doorway of one of the bedrooms where Marianne happened to be tidying up. She caught a glimpse of Colin as I led him by and instantly read the signals.

"I'll make you both some coffee," she said, and immediately slipped back into the kitchen.

I directed Colin to the most comfortable chair in my study; the leather one at my desk. I turned it around for him and pulled up another chair beside it. He sat down, his elbows on its padded arms, supporting his head in his hands.

"Colin, what's wrong?" I asked softly, putting my arm around him. I knew from the little shudder I felt in his shoulder and the sharp intake of his breath, that he was about to cry.

I waited until he was ready to speak.

"It's my mother," he sobbed, "she's just passed away."

In that instant, I thought I detected in his blue-green eyes something other than the brimming tears of sorrow and loss.

It was, perhaps, a gentle glint of joy. Could it be that his mother had become a believer before she died? I never was totally certain; only God knows for sure. However, it is certain that Colin and his mother did become reconciled to each other in this life.

"Oh, Marcus," he said, his voice laden with emotion, "I'm so glad that God gave my mother back to me!"

I squeezed his hand in a reassuring grip.

He gave my hand a reciprocal squeeze. Then he smiled.

When Colin, who'd never known his father, trusted Christ, he found for the first time the security and love of a real father—the Lord God of Heaven. And once he'd begun to put things right in his life, his Heavenly Father graciously restored his earthly mother to him.

At last, Colin knew what it really meant to belong to a family.

Room 105

Chapter 14

Because of highly motivated people like Colin and Steve, the Camdenville ministry, in Newtown Parish, began to show unmistakable signs of healthy spiritual growth. Whilst there were always down-and-outs to feed, clothe, and physically care for, Marianne and I were grateful for the personnel the Lord raised up to help us meet the spiritual needs of the work. God began to lay solid foundations through the faithful commitment of these people in Sunday school, youth groups, the Saturday street and coffee shop outreach and our Sunday services—especially the monthly evangelistic ones.

By 1977 the little Camdenville Chapel was too small for our meetings. So the people of the fellowship began to renovate the old church hall next door. Colin, who was always there when work was to be done, was in his element. At almost any hour of the day or night, one was likely to find him in the hall, often with others, but frequently alone, busily sawing, hammering or painting.

Steve, like Colin, was also keen to help us meet any one of a wide range of church needs. We appointed him our church bus driver—a role he fulfilled with great efficiency and reliability. Not only did he transport our inner-city young people to the youth meetings, where they joined with busloads of others from Greater Metropolitan Sydney, but he rarely missed an opportunity to invite anyone he met to come and hear the gospel preached.

Some time after this, Steve invited a tall young blonde woman, named Helen, to church. She came to our evening service and afterwards stayed back, as many used to do, to have a cup of tea and to talk.

Steve, who was very sensitive to people's problems, discerned that Helen was under some kind of heavy burden. So he introduced her to Marianne and the two were soon engaged in conversation. Marianne discovered that Helen had originally come from Coffs Harbour, which gave them some common discussion ground. But she was unable to discover what Helen's problem was. Helen simply refused to open up to her.

A few weeks later, at 3:00 o'clock on a Monday morning, our front door-bell rang.

I hurriedly donned my dressing gown and went to see who it was.

It was Helen. I remembered her from her visit to our church.

"Pastor Luedi," she said with some effort, her speech slow and labored, her eyes heavy-lidded "...can I speak to Marianne?"

"Come inside, Helen," I said. I took her into our living room.

I asked her to sit down and went back to our bedroom to tell Marianne.

As I entered, Marianne reached across and switched on the bed lamp. Shielding her squinting eyes from its brightness, she sleepily asked,

"Who was that at the door?"

"It's Helen," I said quietly, "...the young woman you spoke with after church a few weeks ago."

"What does she want?"

"I don't know," I replied softly, "but she's asked to talk to you."

As Marianne climbed out of bed, I helped her on with her dressing gown.

"She's been on drugs, darling," I whispered. "She's stoned. I left her in the living room. Why don't you talk to her for a while? I'll be here if you need me."

"Okay darling, I'll do my best," she said as she put on her slippers and knotted the tie of her gown.

Within 10 minutes Marianne was back.

"I think you'd better come and talk to her, dear," she said.

I went with Marianne into the living room.

Helen was sitting there motionless, her hand to her forehead, just staring blankly at the floor. Marianne sat beside her. Then, taking her hand she said to me, "Darling, Helen drove her car here this morning—she's high on drugs—how she made it alive, I don't know. But she was desperate to talk to someone about the trouble she's in."

Marianne looked back at Helen and waited for her to speak. She said nothing, so Marianne continued. "Helen has just told me that for the past two years she has been living a double life. By day she's the respectable housewife with two children, but by night, she's a prostitute in King's Cross.

"She's been doing this now for two years. And her husband, who's a mail man on Sydney's North shore, has no idea that this has been going on. In fact, he thought she'd been working all this time as a night-club entertainer."

As Marianne recounted all this, Helen did not react in any way.

"Helen," I asked, "why did you do this? Why do you work as a prostitute?"

"I have to," she replied, her words expressionless and elongated, "...gotta pay the bills...I'm hooked on heroin, too...gotta support that as well."

Helen's predicament called for immediate and radical attention.

"Helen," I said, "Marianne is going to get us all a cup of coffee. After that, I'm going to drive you to your home. As soon as we get there, I'm going to wake your husband. And you're going to tell him exactly what you've told us here, this morning. Do you understand?"

"Yes," she said dully.

"Are you willing to do that—to tell your husband that you've been a prostitute for the last two years?"

"Yes," she said again.

I got dressed while Marianne made the coffee.

In 10 minutes Helen and I were on our way.

In half an hour we'd arrived at the house where she lived with her husband and their two children. She unlocked the front door and immediately walked towards their bedroom. I followed her. When she opened the door, I could see her husband asleep in the bed. She went in and shook him.

"Jason, wake up...someone wants to talk to you!"

"What's wrong?" he cried, throwing back the blankets and almost leaping out of bed.

He stood there, with nothing on but his shorts, trying to make out who I was.

I put my hand on his shoulder and said, as calmly as I could,

"I'm Marcus Luedi, Jason. I'm a Pastor of the Newtown Church. Helen and I need to talk to you."

Still only half awake, he fumbled through the clothes in his wardrobe until he found his dressing gown.

We all went into the adjacent living room and sat down.

"Helen has something to tell you, Jason," I said.

"What is it?" he asked urgently.

Helen did not speak.

"What is it?" he asked again, sensing that we must have had some very bad news for him.

It was clear that Helen would not, or could not, bring herself to tell her husband what she'd been doing. And it was also clear that he was totally unaware of her involvement in either prostitution or drugs. I knew that the unpleasant task of telling this poor fellow the truth was now mine.

Slowly and carefully I explained the situation to him.

His immediate reaction was one of utter disbelief.

"It can't be true," he gasped. "Helen, is this true?"

"Yes," she murmured flatly.

For the next half hour I felt like an inexperienced lifeguard who'd been suddenly called upon to bring a drowning man to shore through the pounding surf. As successive waves of horror, anger and shattering helplessness crashed over him, I could do little more than keep him afloat.

I realized, however, in spite of my own feelings of impotence and frustration, that God could, and would, salvage Helen's and Jason's relationship, if each of them would unconditionally hand over their lives to Him.

I made arrangements for both of them to come that week to receive spiritual counsel and ongoing support from the church. They did this and there were soon indications that God was beginning to work in their lives. Helen left prostitution and three weeks later, to our delight, was led to Christ by the man who first brought her to our church—Steve.

We also took steps to get her into a program where her drug problem could be treated. Whilst there were agencies doing this kind of work around Sydney, I saw the need for people like Helen, to be placed in a Christian drug rehabilitation program; one that operated on a thoroughly biblical basis. It needed, I believed, to be in some place that was far away from the city and its allurements, a place where a godly and experienced staff would lead drug addicts, and perhaps alcohol addicts as well, to Christ. Then, in the power which God would provide through His Holy Spirit, these people could be properly, and hopefully, rehabilitated—permanently.

How pleased I was when I learned that my friend Jean-Pierre had recently returned to Coffs Harbour to establish exactly this kind of program.

Late in 1977 he phoned me about it, then, to my great surprise, told me he'd just bought a 130-acre property in the mountains some 20 or so miles from Coffs Harbour. Shortly after this, Marianne, the girls and I went back to Coffs Harbour for our Christmas vacation. Of course Jean-Pierre and Honi were keen to show the site to us while we were there.

So, about 10 o'clock one hot December morning, they picked us up in their four-wheel-drive Land Rover to take us there.

"Would you believe it," said Jean-Pierre, as we drove out of the town, "when we sold our house in Western Australia, we had just enough money to buy this land and a couple of slashers to cut down the grass?"

"It's called *Sherwood Cliffs*," he added.

"Are there any buildings on it?" I asked.

"No," he replied. "Apart from the fences around it and a rough track through it, it's pretty much the way the Lord created it."

The road we were on was, like most of the roads through this mountain forest region, narrow, unpaved and rough. When we reached the top of the range, all we could see ahead was ridge after ridge of tree-covered mountains. After a few more minutes of driving, a glorious valley opened up below us. On its undulating green floor stood dozens of stark white dead trees. Some of them were 200 feet high. They'd been ring-barked many years ago by the dairy farmer who owned the property at that time.

On the far side of the valley, the perpendicular sandstone cliffs, that gave the place its name, towered hundreds of feet above the forest-covered foothills.

To reach the parcel of land he'd bought on these foothills, Jean-Pierre had first to drive us to the other side of a mountain stream. It was almost overgrown with a canopy of low scrub and blossoming lantana. We bumped our way up the deeply rutted track on the other side until we could proceed no further.

And there, high above us, at the base of the great gray-fawn cliff-face, stood the tall trees of a magnificent virgin rain forest. There were huge strangulum figs, their great buttress-roots locking massive boulders in a permanent embrace. There were lofty flood gums, bloodwoods and tallow-woods, their trunks adorned with curtsying green bouquets of giant elkhorns. Jungle vines and creepers dangled lazily from their branches. And below all this, flourished a lush lower tier of glossy green palms and gracefully fronded tree-ferns.

As we stood there on the edge of this forest, then looked out over this lovely valley, Jean-Pierre and Honi told us of their plans.

In addition to the spiritual therapy that was to be the foundation of their ministry, they envisioned the practical therapy of a self-supporting farm, with its own beef and dairy cattle, crops, fruit orchards and honey. Neither of them seemed daunted by the fact that none of these things had yet been established. Nor did they appear to be concerned that there were no accommodations, no lighting, no power, no telephone and no proper water supply. Furthermore, at this stage, they had no money to finance the project, no staff to run it—and nobody to rehabilitate.

But they were convinced that God was in it and would soon make their dream a reality.

We promised to pray for them, although we were at a loss to understand how God would make it all happen.

Not long after we had returned to Newtown, I received a phone call from Jean-Pierre's father. He and his wife had recently come from Switzerland to visit Jean-Pierre and wanted to spend a brief time with us before flying home.

As soon as they came into our home, I could see that something was troubling them. It was the Sherwood Cliffs project.

"Marcus," said Jean-Pierre's father, "we've just been to see the property our son has bought. I think he's gone mad. Anyone who would sink all his money into a place like that would have to be crazy! Its miles from anywhere, there's nothing on it but trees and rocks!

"When I first heard that Jean-Pierre had bought some land here, I thought I might be able to help him financially to develop it, you know.

"But now," he continued angrily, "now that I've seen it, there's no way I'd ever consider putting a cent towards it. And as for this hair-brained idea he's got of helping alcoholics and drug addicts...that will be a disaster! The whole thing's insane!

"Marcus, you're his friend. Can't you talk him out of it?"

Room 105

Chapter 15

O ur ministry at Camdenville continued to grow, not only numerically, but spiritually. God touched and changed numerous lives. The vibrant faith of people such as Colin, Steve and Peter, was infectious and through them we had the joy of seeing many needy people brought to new life in Christ.

Of course, we still had the ever-continuing problem of derelicts who staggered from crisis to crisis only to find the next meal, the next drink or a place to sleep the next night. Sadly, few of them received the gospel. Of course, most of them readily received everything we offered to save them from *physical* disaster or even death, but few readily received the gift of *spiritual* life which God offered through His Son the Lord Jesus Christ.

How sad it was to see such people continue to reject the gospel, which is the power of God unto salvation to everyone that believes. And how much sadder to see their ungodly attitudes and behaviors inherited by their children. This sad process was exemplified in no-one more graphically than Kathie.

Kathie's own alcohol-dominated existence, and that of George, too, continued without change for as long as we knew them. But even more terrible was the effect of their lives on Kathie's children, especially her daughter, Germaine.

By the time Germaine had reached adulthood, she was already addicted to heroin and was living with a man to whom she had borne a daughter. When I first met her, she was struggling unsuccessfully to raise this little baby by herself, because the father was in jail, convicted of murder.

One night at 11 o'clock, Germaine phoned and begged me to bring food for her baby, Elizabeth. The next morning I picked up some powdered milk from the Mission Store and went to her house.

When I arrived there, the front door was wide open. I could hear a baby crying inside. I also heard a cat howling, almost as loudly, as though it too was hungry.

"It's Pastor Luedi!" I called out as I knocked on the door frame.

"Come in," Germaine called back, her voice betraying the effect of drugs that was now so familiar to me.

Germaine, a very attractive little 21-year-old, fine-boned and delicate, was lying in a trance-like state on the couch in her living room. The place reeked of urine. On the carpet in a wooden play-pen was her tiny, 12-month-old baby. She lay there in her soaking diaper, her little arms waving as she screamed convulsively.

"I know you're hungry, darling," I said. "I won't be long."

I went into the little kitchen and, as best I could, prepared some warm milk for her and returned with it in a bottle. I had some left over, so I gave it to the cat. When I left Germaine that morning, I did not know that this was to be the last time I would see her alive.

Within 12 months, she was dead. It was her mother, Kathie, who broke the sad news to me.

"She's dead!" Kathie sobbed hysterically. "Pastor Luedi, my lovely daughter is dead! They want me to go and identify her body...I don't think I can do it.... Will you come with me?"

"Of course, Kathie," I said.

Later that day I drove her to the City Morgue. As soon as we went inside, Kathie became hysterical. The policeman on duty there, when he saw the state she was in, took me aside and had a brief word with me. Then he said to Kathie, "Madam, I think you should stay here. Pastor Luedi will complete the identification for us."

I sat Kathie down and tried to pacify her. After a few minutes I was introduced to a middle-aged man in a white lab coat. He wore a plastic-covered name-tag with a colored photograph of himself on it. Against his chest he held a small board on which was clipped a sheaf of official-looking documents.

"Please come this way, Pastor," he said. I followed him down a steel spiral-staircase into a sort of large concrete-floored basement. The place had a curiously sweet smell to it. It reminded me of a gymnasium locker room, except instead of rows of metal cupboards it had four tiers of stainless-steel drawers on either side. The man in the white coat flipped through his notes.

"Oh yes," he said, having located the one he wanted. "Number 37."

We walked together to the drawer with that number on it. Gently he pulled it partly open, as one does the drawer of a filing cabinet. And there she was; poor Germaine, so motionless and silent, her little body clothed in a short white gown; her dainty face still lovely—even in death.

"That's Germaine," I said.

Once the necessary documents had been signed, I took Kathie back home. When we arrived, she was still quite distraught, so I thought it best to go inside and stay with her for a while.

As soon as we opened the front door, Germaine's little two-year-old daughter, Elizabeth, who'd been left with George, came running to meet us.

"Where's my mummy?" she cried.

The words nearly broke my heart. I took her tiny body in my arms. As I held her, I wondered what kind of life *her* children would have—if she survived to bear them.

There seemed to be some dark, hereditary influence at work in this family. Having come down from an alcoholic grandmother, it had expressed itself in the tragic life and death of her heroin-addicted daughter, and would almost certainly emerge in some equally destructive form in the granddaughter—unless the wretched process were somehow broken.

I was convinced that only the power of God in Christ could do this. And if it did not, then God would continue to bring His judgment upon the family through the inheritance of their ungodliness, exactly as He Himself said He would, "...*visiting the iniquity of the fathers upon the children of the third and fourth generation of them that hate me*" (Exodus 20:5).

Hopeless as this whole situation seemed, God once more was about to bring something good out of it. This began at Germaine's funeral, where I noticed a young man who seemed particularly distressed. When the burial service was over, he sought me out.

"I'm Robert," he said, limply shaking my hand. "I was living with Germaine before she died.... I loved her, Pastor. I really did, and I loved her little daughter as well. But now that Germaine is dead, I just want to die too. I have nothing to live for."

I suspected, from the way he talked, that this well-dressed young man was very possibly a drug addict too. In his present state of mind, I could see him being suicidal.

"Robert," I said, "don't talk like that. In spite of what's happened and, regardless of the way you feel right now, your life can be given meaning—real meaning if you truly desire it."

"I'd like to talk further with you," I added, as Marianne came and stood by my side. "Why don't you come to our parsonage at Camdenville to discuss things? I'd really like to help you."

"Perhaps you'd like to have dinner with us," said Marianne.

"How about Tuesday night?" I suggested.

"Okay," he replied, "I'll come."

And he did, the following Tuesday, our guest night. That evening, we did our best to make him feel we cared for him. Just before he left, we invited him to join our Camdenville fellowship.

The following Sunday night he was there. He seemed to sense right away that he was not the only person there with problems. There were many who, like himself, were seeking help; people with drug problems, alcoholics, prostitutes, even a woman who earlier had been a witch. Robert realized that there were people present, who, as converted Christians, were now happy and able to control their problems, as well as help others to do the same.

Robert felt relaxed and accepted that night and, when we talked with him over a cup of tea, he started to open up. As I had suspected, he did have a drug problem. Like Germaine, he too was a heroin addict.

The following week, Robert was arrested for possession of drugs and taken into custody. They held him there for three weeks prior to his trial. While Robert was in jail, I began to give some thought as to what steps might be taken to rehabilitate him.

I decided, as a first step, to give him a copy of a book by David Wilkerson entitled *Run, Baby, Run* which described how a drug addict, through the power of God, conquered his habit. I gave him a copy of this book when I next visited him. He accepted it gratefully and promised to read it.

My next step was to phone Jean-Pierre whose work at Sherwood Cliffs had now started to move forward. Jean-Pierre had limited accommodations on his property, in the form of four railway cars. His friend, John Smith, owner of an engineering company, had transported them to the site, with great difficulty, using one of his large semi-trailers. This enabled Jean-Pierre to launch his rehabilitation program, starting with two alcoholics.

I told Jean-Pierre about Robert and, although I could not predict the outcome of his forthcoming trial, asked Jean-Pierre whether he would be willing to take him, at Sherwood Cliffs, if it could be arranged. He said he would.

As we had all expected, Robert was found guilty as charged.

The judge placed him on a three-year bond, conditional on his receiving drug rehabilitation. Robert's lawyer, at my suggestion, requested that he be sent to Sherwood Cliffs to enter Jean-Pierre's program there. Although the judge was told that this program had barely begun and as yet had no proven track record, he agreed to the arrangement and Robert became Sherwood Cliffs' first heroin addict.

I was much encouraged by this, and all the more so because Robert himself was keen to go. Having read the book which I had given him, he told me that he now sincerely desired to lay hold of those spiritual resources available in Christ, that he might be set free from his addiction.

Robert's going to Sherwood Cliffs marked the beginning of a joint ministry which Jean-Pierre and I were to share over subsequent years.

Jean-Pierre's rehabilitation program soon emerged as the ideal place to send people we were not equipped to handle in Newtown. I was confident that his Sherwood Cliffs program would eventually become one of the most successful rehabilitation ventures in the country. The fact that everybody was presently accommodated in four railway carriages and a leaky old bus, did not dampen the enthusiasm of any of those exercising or receiving this ministry. The foundations for the buildings of a small village, with its own water and power supply, would soon be laid. However, the real foundations for the work to be done at Sherwood Cliffs were not of bricks and mortar. They were of another kind. Jean-Pierre, Honi and the others who labored with them, were convinced that the work there had to be built on the principles of God's Word, the Bible. Those who came for help would also need to understand that, unless they too were willing to build on this foundation, there would be no real rehabilitation for them. And this would only happen as the gospel was faithfully preached to them and they responded scripturally with true repentance and faith, trusting Christ as Savior and Lord: *"For other foundation can no man lay than that which is laid, which is Jesus Christ"* (1 Corinthians 3:11).

All those who came into the program were told that they were embarking on a spiritual quest, a personal quest to find Christ, and the sin-conquering power of His life. For this reason they would be known throughout their stay at Sherwood Cliffs as "seekers."

Jean-Pierre and his co-workers made it clear from the outset that if a man found salvation through the divine power of God, then the power of that same God was more than sufficient to enable his addiction to be broken completely—and permanently. True trust in Christ would bring true freedom.

There was no place at Sherwood Cliffs for the gradual weaning process advocated in so many other rehabilitation institutions. Nor was there any credence given to the theory of replacement therapy; whereby, for example, a heroin addict would go on to a methadone program to ease the trauma of withdrawal. Furthermore, lest one kind of addiction be replaced by another, all seekers were told that smoking was banned—and not only for them, as inmates, but for all those on staff and everyone who came onto the site, including visitors. A notice on the entrance gate made this position absolutely clear.

Sherwood Cliffs' *cold turkey* policy, because it was so radically different to that employed in most other programs, was often roundly criticized as inhuman, even cruel. This opinion was not shared by either seekers or staff. Their success rate spoke for itself. For example, whereas the officially claimed success rate for heroin addicts treated in government institutions was 2% to 5%, at Sherwood Cliffs it was a staggering 70%.

Jean-Pierre realized from the very beginning, that the work could not be really effective without a dedicated Christian staff, at least equal in numbers to the seekers. Only with such a ratio would it be possible, he claimed, to firmly, but lovingly and patiently apply, on an individual basis, the necessary spiritual principles and disciplines needed.

The Sherwood Cliffs foundational reliance upon Scripture gave rise to another principle which was laid down early in its operation. If God's miraculous rehabilitation work was to be done in God's way, then that work would need to be free and autonomous to do it. For this reason, a firm decision was made never to accept any form of government funding with its inevitable danger of ultimate government control.

Few, who witnessed the early years of this unconventional Christian ministry, would have expected that God would bless it and establish it as one of the most successful rehabilitation works operating anywhere in the world.

During the next few years, while Jean-Pierre's ministry at Sherwood Cliffs began to expand, my ministry at Newtown began to draw to a close.

By 1979, Marianne and I had been at Newtown for over four years. Although they were heavy and difficult years, they had been wonderfully blessed by God. However, around this time, I became increasingly aware of factors that caused me to assess the wisdom of continuing on in this inner-city ministry.

One of these factors concerned the nature of the ministry itself and certain changes which had begun to occur. A change in parish leadership had brought with it a marked difference in the kind and quality of outreach in the mission. The Camdenville services were stopped and the congregation was asked to attend the large Newtown church. As a result of this, the Camdenville people suddenly found themselves in a setting where they felt they did not belong. The numbers worshipping there were certainly larger but the intimacy was gone. Our people had lost their identity.

But I feared they were in danger of losing much more than this. Would this heavy emphasis on bigger numbers bring with it a loss of the doctrinal emphasis, which had come to characterize the Camdenville ministry and its people? And was there not a danger that the simple but dynamically scriptural faith of our little congregation might be lost in the large numbers of people swept along in an impressive, but superficial, religious experience?

As a committed Bible preacher, I seriously began to wonder whether I could continue to function in a context where such trends were emerging.

The second factor, that caused me to consider the wisdom of continuing at Newtown, was my growing desire to exercise a rural-based ministry to young people who were caught in the problems of increasingly widespread unemployment. Like Jean-Pierre, I felt that such a ministry could best be exercised on a faith basis that was organizationally independent and outside the framework of denominational control.

There was a third factor, perhaps the major one, which suggested that it might be time to terminate my Newtown ministry. It concerned my family. Marianne was due to give birth to our fourth child in August of that year. And I had noticed that, as her pregnancy continued, she found it increasingly difficult to cope with the stresses which our ministry imposed. I noticed particularly that she tended to become quite upset when she sensed that people were taking advantage of me, and were thereby placing undue strain, not only on me, but on everyone in our family.

Her highly stressed state of mind was clearly evidenced, one morning just after midnight, when Kathie rang our front door-bell and called out in a voice slurred by alcohol, "Pastor, Pastor, please help me!" Unannounced visits from Kathie were by no means unusual but, as I sat up in bed, I wondered what she could possibly want at this unearthly hour. Before my finger had even found the switch on our bed lamp, I felt Marianne's hand on my arm. She held it in a firm grip.

"Marcus," she said, in a low, determined voice, "It's Kathie again...I've told you many times—she's only using you."

"I know that, darling," I whispered in reply, "but she seems to be in some kind of trouble...it's my ministry to help her!"

"Marcus," Marianne said, with even more deliberation, "you are not to go to that door...I mean it! If you do, I'll divorce you!"

I realized of course that Marianne would never contemplate, let alone do such a thing, but that her angry threat was an expression of the emotional stress this situation had triggered off.

"Pastor, Pastor!" shouted Kathie as she rang our door-bell again then rapped noisily on the door. "I know you're in there! Help me, I'm in pain!"

"Marianne," I whispered with urgency, "I've got to find out what's wrong."

"Marcus," she cut in with an almost venomous whisper, "I've had enough and I'm putting my foot down this time! You are not to go out to her!"

I lay there motionless, in reluctant tight-lipped silence, as Kathie continued to hammer on our door. "Open the door, Pastor," she whined, "I'm in terrific pain!"

Even in the darkness, I could feel the intensity of Marianne's implacable anger. In that moment, I realized that my wife was not only fiercely protecting her husband from being used by a thoughtless and irresponsible woman, but was making a last ditch stand to defend her family.

I knew I was no match for her while she was in this frame of mind. So with great difficulty, I stifled my conscience and lay there, while Kathie continued to shout and batter on our door.

Eventually there was a pause, then a torrent of vile abuse and swearing. After a few brief moments of silence, we heard the sound of departing footsteps.

Marianne's grip on my arm tightened—a warning to me not to relent.

When all was again silent, I peered cautiously out between the curtains. To my surprise, there was Kathie on the other side of the road. She had gone across to the Roman Catholic rectory there.

"She's knocking on Father Brien's door," I said.

In an instant Marianne was kneeling on the bed beside me, her face next to mine. With mouths agape, we watched the front light go on and saw the priest come out and take Kathie inside, closing the door behind him.

I was stunned by all this and lay back on the bed, staring up into the darkness of our bedroom. This was the first time in my entire ministry I'd not responded to someone who had sought my help. And now the person to whom I'd refused that help had sought it from a Roman Catholic priest.

Marianne lay down beside me.

Neither of us spoke.

It was impossible to verbalize the self-condemnation we both felt; Marianne for having forbidden me to help Kathie, and I for obeying her. Terrible as these feelings were, they were soon to become even worse.

In barely five minutes, an ambulance pulled up across the road, its red light rhythmically turning. Two ambulance officers knocked on the rectory door. We saw them take a stretcher inside and, in mute horror, watched them wheel Kathie out and place her in the ambulance.

When it was all over, I sat on the edge of the bed, my head in my hands. "I feel I have failed my ministry," I said with shame.

Marianne said nothing.

Neither of us slept that night.

That morning at the hospital, I was told that Kathie had been admitted as an emergency case. George, in a drunken frenzy, had beaten her about the head, then brutally kicked her in the lower back, rupturing a kidney.

What could I say to her as she lay there in the recovery ward, her face swollen and her eyes two dark slits?

Here was a woman, who, when she came to me earlier that morning, was seriously injured and internally hemorrhaging. She could easily have died.

I placed a chair next to her bed and sat down. I reached out to take the hand that lay limply on the cover-sheet. I hesitated, as it suddenly occurred to me, that this was the same hand that only a few hours ago, had been stretched forth for my help—and been rejected.

This was the hand which, when clenched by pain into an angry fist, had beaten frantically on my door—and been ignored.

"Kathie," I said, closing my eyes and trying hard to choose the words that I knew could never express the regret and self-loathing I felt, "Kathie...I am sorry. I'm sorry I didn't respond to your cry for help early this morning. I know now that you were in deep trouble...that it was a serious crisis for you.

"But Kathie," I went on, taking her hand and looking earnestly into those eyes that were almost swollen shut, "Marianne and I had reached a crisis point in our lives too! When you came to our home this morning, Marianne became very upset. She said that, for years now, you have been using me. And she was perfectly right. That is exactly what you have been doing—and this has put heavy strain, not only on me, but on my whole family. She told me that she'd had enough of it and forbade me to go out to you. Against my better judgment, I decided not to help you. I know now that I was wrong. We both were, and I want to apologize."

This experience had a sobering effect upon the three of us. God used it to enlighten us all concerning the true nature of my ministry and its responsibilities. But for me, as a husband and father, it was a critically important learning experience. I realized, as never before, that the *total availability* course I had adopted, throughout my ministry, had placed burdens upon my precious wife and family which they could not handle and should never have been called upon to bear.

As I took these three factors into account, then discussed them and prayed about them with Marianne, I decided that, having completed nearly five years at Newtown, I ought to hand in my resignation as a Uniting Church pastor there and seek a ministry to unemployed young people in the rural setting near Coffs Harbour.

The Board of Missions accepted my resignation. The General Secretary responded with a warm letter, in which he expressed his personal gratitude for my service and commitment as a pastor. He went on to assure me of his continued prayerful support and friendship, as I moved, with my family, into a new phase of Christian service.

In July, 1979, we returned to Coffs Harbour, where we were sure that our lives would be far less stressful than they had been in Sydney.

We were soon to find out just how wrong we were about this.

Room
105

Chapter 16

"For as the heavens are higher than the earth, so are my ways higher than your ways and my thoughts higher than your thoughts. For my thoughts are not your thoughts, neither are your ways my ways, saith the Lord" (Isaiah 55:8,9).

God was about to teach us this lesson during our time in Coffs Harbour.

We thought we knew the best ways to serve Him and had made careful plans to put them into operation. But God had other thoughts, other ways and other means by which He would prepare and use us. It would be only after years of the most excruciating hardship and suffering, that God would begin to reveal what He was doing, how He was doing it, and ultimately, why.

Upon our return to Coffs Harbour, we moved into a house provided by a Christian friend named Paul Wagner, who shared our vision for the independent work with unemployed young people we had come back to establish. Marianne and I were especially pleased to have Paul's house to live in because, only a few weeks after our arrival, our little son was born. We called him Andrew.

Paul also arranged for me to manage and work a banana plantation he had acquired just out of town; the idea being that, while I did this, I would be able to look for a property suitable for our ministry.

Unfortunately, after a year of continuous searching, we had not been successful in acquiring such a property. Consequently, our ministry, which we had decided to call *Bethany*, could not operate as planned, unless such land were available.

Towards the latter part of 1980, an opportunity for me to work with young people did in fact emerge, but not as I had envisaged it. The Parish Council of the Coffs Harbour Uniting Church invited me to take up the newly created position of Youth Director for the district. However, because of my intention to inaugurate our *Bethany* ministry, I told them I would be willing to take the position only for 12 months. They agreed to my conditions and I accepted the post. Although God blessed this ministry, Marianne and I saw it essentially as a step towards our independent *Bethany* project, and as the year drew to a close, we began to look forward to it with eager anticipation.

Early in the new year of 1982, Claudia went to Sydney to begin training as a nurse.

It was around this time that an urgent Parish need suddenly arose. Two full-time leadership positions were unexpectedly made vacant in the area and I was approached to fill one of them—that of minister at Sawtell, a southern beach-side suburb of Coffs Harbour. I told them that, since it was an emergency, I would be willing to take the position, but as before, only for 12 months. Once again, I was accepted on this basis, and, after that year was ended in January of 1983, a property, suitable for our purpose, became available on the outskirts of Coffs Harbour.

Bethany was designed to function as an independent Christian co-operative ministry to unemployed young people, who, by engaging in market-gardening and related activities, would be fitted to take their place in society as skilled and responsible Christian citizens.

Within a month, the ministry was operational, starting with five young men. At last we were underway and free to pursue our vision, or so we thought.

However, what in fact happened was that the ministry, although it grew and began to achieve its stated aims, was constantly under the threat of being undermined by ongoing property problems. Because of these problems, the entire operation had to be relocated three times in as many years. In this harrowing process, Marianne and I had put all our money into the venture, and had lost everything. Others had lost a great deal of their money too.

During this difficult time, I was assisted financially by the Baptist Church in Coffs Harbour as I fulfilled, on a part-time basis with them, the role of Assistant Pastor.

At this time, our second daughter, Sandra, went to Sydney where she enrolled in a child care course. With our two teenage daughters now studying in the city, we were a much smaller family, with only two children; Natasha, 11, and Andrew, five.

One Sunday morning, during a worship service there, my attention was drawn to the church motto, written in gold letters on the wall behind the pulpit. It read: '*To be molded into the image of Christ.*' As I looked at these words I found myself thinking, "That's what I want...that's what I need."

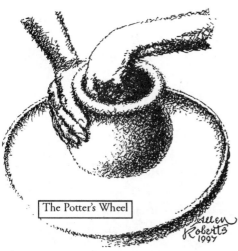

The Potter's Wheel

Then, silently and fervently, I prayed, "Lord, mold *me*. Make me what *You* want me to be— that I might be effective in whatever ministry You have for me."

I knew that God, as the divine potter, described in such passages as Isaiah 64:8 and Romans 9:21, was already working on me. And I knew that the process had already involved some painful 'pummeling'. But I was also acutely aware that, if I were to be a useful vessel in His hands, there was much more to come. How much more, I was shortly to discover.

In January, 1986, *Bethany* was again re-established, this time on a 12-acre property with the curiously significant name of *Potter's Nursery.*

To begin with, the ministry went very well indeed. We soon had 10 young men working the nursery and establishing a commercial-garden on the property. In the first three months, our productivity increased by 25%. But the most pleasing aspect of the work was the spiritual growth, fostered through our daily Bible studies and prayer times.

At this time, the Boyces, a dedicated Christian family, came and

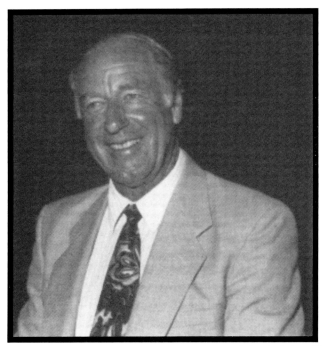

This is me, Marcus Luedi.

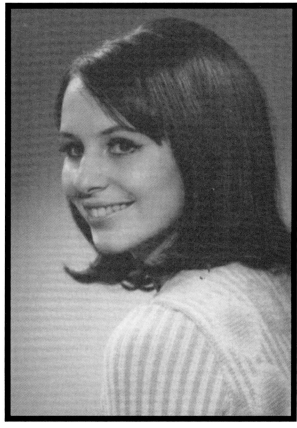

My wife, Marianne, in 1968 as a young woman. Do you see why she got that movie offer? *I* certainly do!

Andrew at 11 years of age, having recovered from his brain-tumor operation.

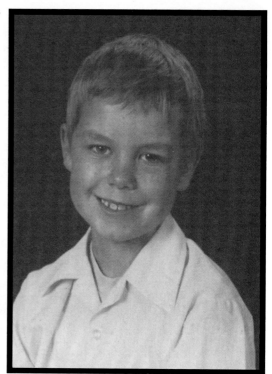

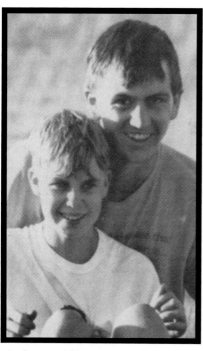

Andrew and his Camp Quality counselor, Kris, in 1991.

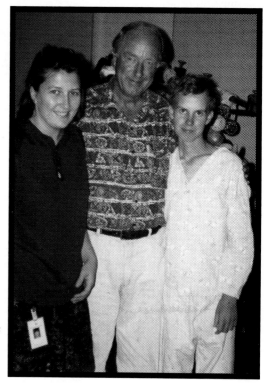

From right, Andrew with me and Tracy in Camperdown Children's Hospital, 1992.

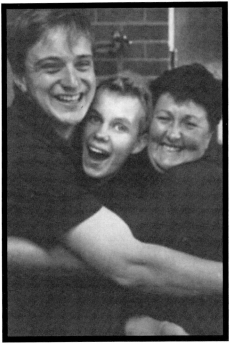

During Andrew's happiest days, at his last Camp Quality, he clowns around with his camp counselor, Matthew, left, and Lisa Hodge, 1993.

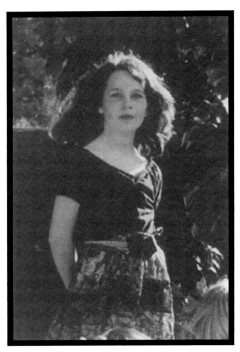

Lisa Augustine (Andrew's roommate at Camperdown Children's Hospital) just prior to her brain-tumor operation.

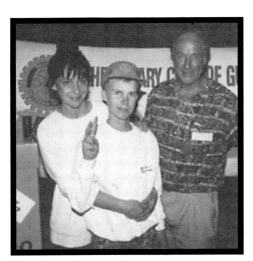

Claudia and I send off Andrew to Disneyland at Sydney Airport, 1993.

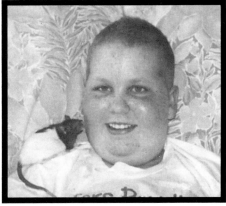

Lisa Augustine shortly before her death, playing with a pet mouse, 1992. You can see the effect of the cancer treatments, puffiness and loss of hair.

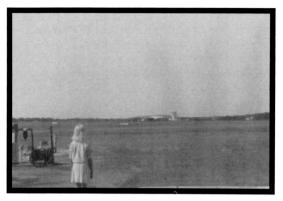

Andrew's sister, Natasha, possibly wondering,
Will I ever see my little brother again?

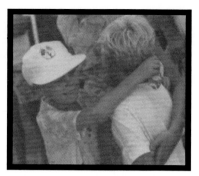

Andrew's pal, Timothy Fox, right,
welcomes Andrew home with a
warm hug following the operation
in 1987.

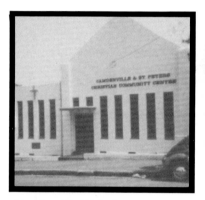

Camdenville Christian
Community Centre, 1976.

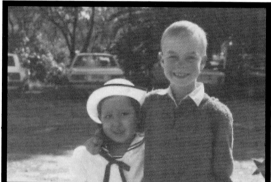

Andrew and his hospital roommate, Ji-Hye, at
Thanksgiving service in Coffs Harbour, 1987.

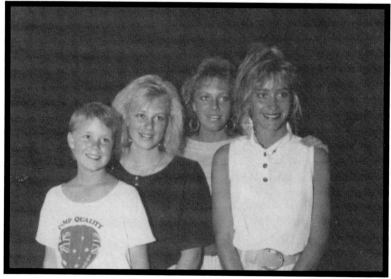

Andrew with his sisters: from left, Natasha, Sandra and Claudia.

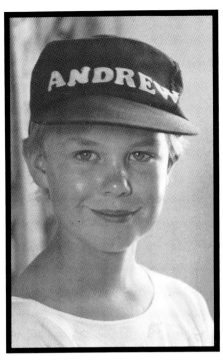

Andrew models his cap, given him at Camp Quality in 1989.

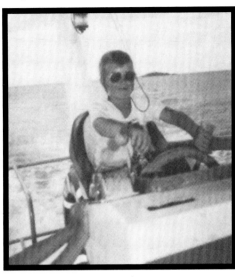

'Captain Andrew' takes the helm of Camp Quality's motor yacht. 1989.

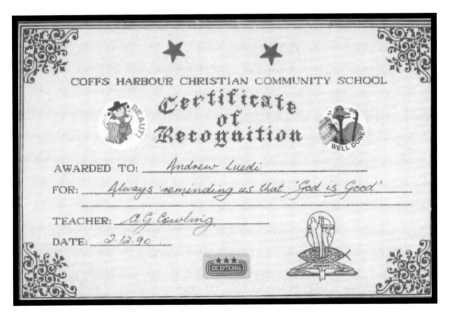

Andrew's certificate of recognition from his school, 1990. You can see by the notation that he was always joyfully witnessing of his sweet relationship with God.

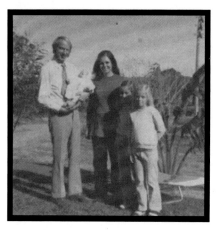

Our family at the birth of Natasha in 1974. From left: me, Natasha, Marianne, Claudia and Sandra.

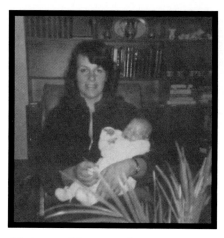

Marianne with our newborn son Andrew, 1979.

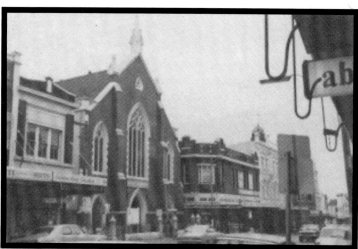

My first pastoral assignment, Newtown Uniting Church Mission in Sydney.

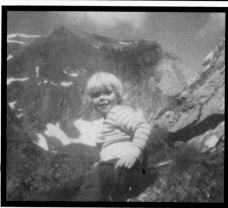

Andrew at age three in the breathtaking Bernese Alps of Switzerland, 1982.

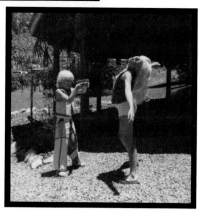

Andrew playing cowboys-and-Indians with his sister Natasha, 1985.

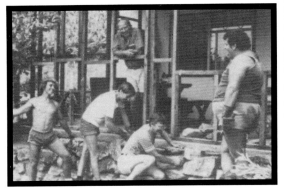

I lean through a roughed-out wall as various members of the *Bethany* ministry renovate our home, 1984.

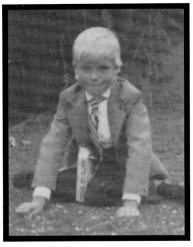

Andrew as a 'page boy' six weeks prior to his first brain-tumor operation, 1986.

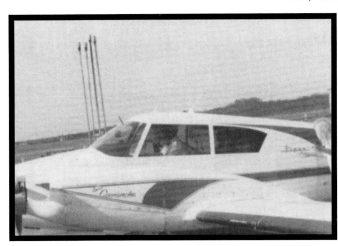

The emergency flight to Sydney for Andrew's first brain-tumor operation, 1986.

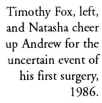

Timothy Fox, left, and Natasha cheer up Andrew for the uncertain event of his first surgery, 1986.

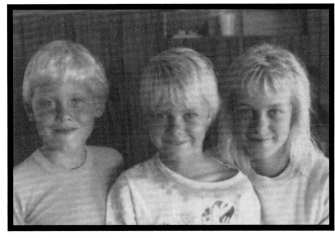

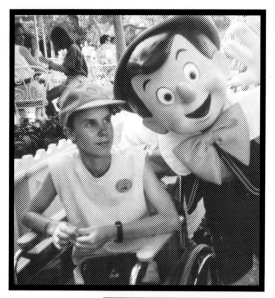

Andrew meets that famous boy, Pinocchio, at Disneyland, just three weeks before his homegoing to Heaven.

Andrew, left, talks with Glenn Smith for the last time, about going to Heaven soon, 1993.

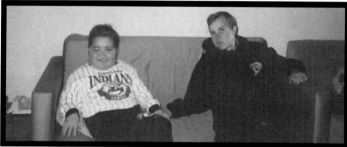

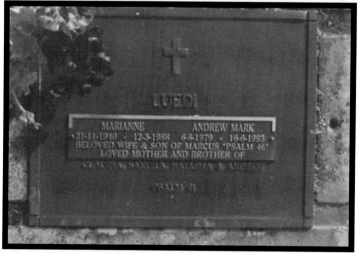

Andrew's body rests with that of his mother in the Lawn Cemetery in Coffs Harbour. We chose Psalm 41 as a theme passage for the grave site, which speaks of our victory in God, even in the face of the death of our mortal bodies. Andrew and Marianne are home at last!

joined the ministry. They also purchased, then brought on site, four large army barracks to accommodate the two families and some workers. As it flourished, the ministry caught the attention of the local newspaper and television media who publicized it widely. By the end of March, that year, everything appeared to be going wonderfully well.

At long last, it seemed, our *Bethany* ministry was firmly established and its future looked bright.

Then, at the beginning of the very next month, ironically at *Potter's Nursery*, the molding process for which I had so earnestly prayed, began.

It was to continue, without abatement, for the ensuing seven years.

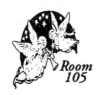
Room 105

Chapter 17

At 2:00 p.m. on Easter Monday, our nursery was struck by a tropical cyclone. Gale-force winds, the worst in a quarter of a century, demolished our glass-house, which contained many thousands of seedlings and young plants. These violent winds also collapsed the large greenhouse which contained our indoor plants and trees.

Immediately after the storm had passed, we all worked hard to stack those plants which had not been damaged into our large shed.

Time prevented us from putting them all under cover and, by sundown, hundreds were dead, shriveled brown by the fierce sub-tropical heat.

The overall damage was extensive and financially ruinous.

Local and national television crews were soon on site filming the destruction for the evening news. Paul Wagner saw it and drove over the next day to discuss the situation with me.

"What do you plan to do, Marcus?" he asked.

"I really don't know," I said. "We simply don't have the resources to repair the damage and become operational again...I'm afraid we're finished, Paul."

"Perhaps there's a way I can help," said Paul. "I've got a friend who's an experienced nurseryman. He's just come down from

Queensland. He lives near me in Nambucca Heads. He's not a Christian, but when I told him about your ministry and the cyclone, he said he'd like to help you get things going again—even offered his services free of charge.

"Why don't we meet with him tomorrow to discuss it?"

I was grateful for Paul's suggestion and, the next day, Marianne and I had a meeting with Paul and his nurseryman friend, whose name was Bill.

Paul had a proposition. It was that Bill become the manager of the nursery. Then, with funds that Paul would donate, Bill would rebuild and restock it, then run it for us. The arrangement, said Paul, would involve Bill being in total charge of the whole nursery and its operation. Of course, the management and development of the garden co-operative would continue to be my responsibility.

Bill reiterated that he was willing to do all this without any payment whatsoever. However, he did say that, since he would be traveling from his home to the nursery and back again each day (a distance of some 60 miles), he would be grateful if he could be reimbursed for the money he would spend on gas.

In view of the fact that Paul's proposal was really the only alternative we had, Marianne and I had to agree that Paul's proposition seemed both feasible and reasonable—even generous.

Nonetheless, I had some reservations.

One of them was, that the autonomy of our ministry, which I had deemed so important, would be reduced markedly by this arrangement. The nursery, which so far had constituted the major part of the work done by our young men, would now come under Bill's control. In establishing *Bethany*, we had sought to be completely independent of governments and even Christian denominations. And now a major part of *Bethany's* operation was about to be placed under the control of one man—and a man who made no profession of being a Christian believer.

I raised this concern with Paul, but he was adamant that his proposition should stand as it was.

I also had some concerns that Bill, since he was not a Christian, would lack the important spiritual insights integral to the ministry and its operation. When this was raised, Bill said he would be perfectly happy to identify with the spiritual aspects of the work and promised to attend our daily Bible study and prayer times.

After our discussion, I still had reservations about the proposition. However, since I was really in no position to bargain, I agreed that a contract should be drawn up on the basis Paul had recommended.

The contract was signed the following day.

As we shook hands on the deal, Bill said to me, "Marcus, just leave everything to me. I'll make this nursery the envy of every nurseryman in this part of the country."

Then, to my dismay, the very next day Bill came to me and said, "Marcus, I've been looking at the costs that I'll have to meet to repair and restock the nursery, and, until everything is running at a profit again, I won't be able to pay you and your family any money to live on."

This jolted me. The meager financial support on which Marianne, the children, and I had been living had come from the profits of the nursery.

"How will we survive?" I asked.

"You'll have to go on to Social Security," he replied. "Don't worry about it. It will only be for a month or two—until the nursery is profitable again."

He seemed oblivious to the disorienting effect this suggestion had on me.

A major objective of *Bethany* was to get our unemployed young people *off* Social Security. Yet here was I, the person heading up the whole ministry, being told I would have to go on to Social Security!

The whole idea was spiritually repugnant to me.

When I told him so, his only response was a facile, "Don't worry about it, Marcus."

Something was definitely not right about this man. I suspected that, in spite of Paul's assurances to the contrary, Bill was not what he appeared to be.

With grave misgivings, I applied for Social Security benefits, trusting that the demoralizing situation would not continue long.

As agreed, Bill began at once to work on repairing the damage done to the nursery and restocking it. The young men and I all worked along with him to get the job done. Paul gave Bill some thousands of dollars to pay the expenses incurred in the process and, in less than a month, the structures the cyclone had demolished were rebuilt and largely restocked with plants.

So within two months, the nursery was basically operational again and business was as good as it had been prior to the cyclone. My gardening co-operative was also going very well. Bill, as he had promised, also attended our daily devotional times.

On the surface, it appeared that Paul's idea, to bring Bill in as manager of the nursery, was a good one.

Personally, I wasn't so sure about this.

After three months had passed, I suggested to Bill that it was time he began to pay Marianne and me a regular amount of money again from the profits of the nursery.

But he would not hear of it, saying that his running expenses were still far too high and that he couldn't afford it yet. He also said that because winter was coming on, sales would be down for several more months, so any financial support for us would be quite out of the question.

It was around this time that I began to have other concerns about Bill.

One day, when I was helping out in the nursery, I noticed a lady customer who was trying to decide whether or not she would buy a particular fruit tree. She went to Bill and asked, "This tree produces fruit twice a year doesn't it?"

"Oh yes, Madam," replied Bill, "indeed it does."

When the lady was out of earshot, I went across to Bill and said, "That tree fruits only once a year. The information you gave that lady was not correct."

"Who cares?" he responded. "You tell 'em what they want to hear."

A little later, Bill did something that caused me to have grave doubts about his self-confessed expertise as a nurseryman.

One afternoon, when we were busily making a special soil mix for the seedlings we regularly sold to our clientele of retailers, Bill came up to us and said, "You don't need to go to all that trouble and expense. All you need to use for those seedlings is river sand."

I could scarcely believe my ears.

"Later this week," he added casually, "we'll drive the truck down to the Orara River and get some."

I was amazed that anyone (least of all an experienced nurseryman) should even suggest such a thing. And, since I could see that he meant to do it, I told Paul about it.

Paul's response was disappointing.

"Bill's had extensive experience as a big nurseryman in Queensland, Marcus. I'm sure he knows what he's doing," he said. "Just do what he says. He's the expert."

Later that week, Bill had us all filling pots and punnets with a mixture that consisted mainly of river sand. We then delivered them to the several retail outlets where we were contracted to water and replace them as they were sold.

Within a week, the sand went hard and every plant stagnated and died.

As a result, the owners and managers of the stores where this happened, simply canceled their contracts with us. In one fell swoop, Bill's absurd procedure had virtually destroyed one of our most dependable and lucrative markets.

When I told him this, he simply said, "It doesn't really matter, Marcus. We were all wasting too much time fiddling around with those seedlings anyway. Let's not bother about them any more. The big money's in trees and shrubs—the exotic stuff. From now on we'll concentrate on that."

I resolved at once to find out whether this man was the big nursery operator he claimed to be. So I made several long-distance phone calls to contacts I had in Queensland. When I asked them what they knew about this man and his huge nursery, none of them was aware of any such nursery owned by a man of that name.

One day, around this time, I heard that a sizeable sum of money owed by the nursery had not been paid. Since Bill was responsible for the payment of all bills, I confronted him on the issue. He said it must have been an oversight of some kind and assured me that he would fix the problem by putting a check in the mail right away.

A week later, he had still not paid the amount. When I told him, he passed it off lightly.

"Don't worry about it," he said, as he leaned back on the chair behind his little office desk.

"I *do* worry about it," I replied with deep concern. "The name of our Christian ministry, and my name too, are at stake here."

I could see, from his somewhat bemused expression, that Bill had no interest in preserving anyone's Christian reputation. So I added, "You also have a legal responsibility to pay money owing to our creditors—the last thing we want is to be involved in a court case."

"A court case," he sarcastically laughed, "No one could afford to take us to court to make us pay a few hundred dollars—they'll just write it off as a bad debt and forget it!

"And if they do get nasty about it," he went on, "we'll just tell them we don't have the money now but we'll pay them what we can when we get it. If we slip them 50 bucks every now and then, there's not a thing they can do about it. Marcus, you worry too much!"

His irresponsible attitude angered me.

"Where's your checkbook?" I demanded.

He could see I meant business and he reached into his brief case and took it out.

I took it from his hand, opened it up and laid it in front of him on his desk.

"I'm not leaving until you write out that check," I said.

I put my pen in his hand and stood over him. I watched him sullenly fill out the details.

"Now sign it," I said.

When he'd done so, he tore out the check and threw it on the desk in front of me.

I picked it up and left.

As I walked outside into the sunshine, I found myself wondering what else this deceptive fellow had been up to since he'd been with us.

It was already clear to me that we'd all made a bad mistake in bringing him in and giving him so much power. If he was actually the kind of man I now suspected him to be, then he was dangerous and could easily destroy our entire ministry.

The unrelieved strain of not only having to work with him, but be subservient to him, without being able to redress the problems he was creating, increased daily. After six months, the stress of the situation was becoming very heavy indeed.

Whilst our ministry had survived that disastrous storm, I could see another storm brewing—one that could be even more devastating than its predecessor.

Room 105

Chapter 18

"Marcus!" Marianne called out, "Andrew's seeing double!" There was urgency in her voice.

I left my tomato picking at once and ran to the house.

Marianne was with Andrew in his bedroom. Her face was filled with unspoken anguish as I came in.

"Darling," I said, "you must take him at once to Dr. Naidoo. Don't bother to phone for an appointment," I said, grabbing our car keys and handing them to her, "—just go!"

Without a word Marianne led Andrew down the front steps and over to our car. I watched as they drove off along our driveway, Marianne, somber-faced at the wheel, and Andrew, the top of his little blonde head just visible above the front passenger door.

This was not the first time Marianne had taken Andrew, for emergency treatment, to Dr. Naidoo, our specialist pediatrician. Only a month before, Dr. Naidoo had examined Andrew when he began to have very severe headaches.

These had begun several weeks after a playground accident in which Andrew had struck his head against a brick wall. The pain had been so intense that it made him scream out at night like some wild animal. X-rays failed to reveal the cause of Andrew's pain and no medication was able to reduce it.

I found myself sighing as I slipped on my garden gloves.

What a year this has been, I thought. *First the cyclone, then the con-*

tinuing threat of our ministry's destruction by Bill's mismanagement or worse—and now this.

"Oh God," I whispered, "help us face this latest challenge, and somehow help Andrew's doctors to diagnose and treat him so he can be made well again!"

Dr. Naidoo, on examining Andrew, immediately arranged a CAT scan for that afternoon.

This time I took him to the radiologist. We arrived there at 3:00 p.m. Although there were several people in the waiting room, I went in with Andrew right away.

As the procedure began, I watched through a little window. The radiologist took some 30 scans, each, I understood, one half millimeter cross-section of Andrew's brain. I watched the images as they came up on the monitor.

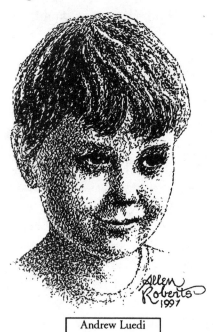

Andrew Luedi

After only 10 minutes or so, the nurse came to me and said, "Mr. Luedi, would you mind going back into the waiting room now please?"

I wondered why she had asked me to leave as I went back and sat down with the other people there. I picked up a magazine and flipped through the first few pages. I had no idea what I was reading.

All I could see was my handsome little seven-year-old son lying there, obediently quiet, in that CAT scan tunnel. And all I could think of was, what they might find and what might happen to this little boy who meant so much to me.

In the last year of hardship, Andrew had been such a joy and encouragement to me. As usual, his school reports had been uniformly excellent. Academically, it seemed, he had a promising future. Would that future be realized now? And what would happen to the strong father-son relationship we had? As often as my heavy schedule permitted over this last year, I had tried hard to spend time with him, even if it were only five or 10 minutes kicking a soccer ball around our back yard. I'd introduced him to fishing and fossicking for gems, both of which he'd come to love as much as I did.

At 3:45 p.m. the radiologist brought Andrew back.

"We've completed the scan, Mr. Luedi," he said. "Would you please wait here with Andrew?"

Andrew sat down next to me as the radiologist went back into his office.

After 30 minutes, I began to wonder why this was taking so long.

After another 30 minutes, I knew something was wrong.

The radiologist did not re-emerge until 5:15 p.m., by which time I was deeply concerned. He held a large yellow envelope in his hand.

"Mr. Luedi," he said, as he handed it to me, "would you please take this to your doctor—at once?"

I glanced at my watch.

"But Dr. Naidoo won't be at his office now," I said, "It's too late."

"No," he responded, "he'll be there, Mr. Luedi—he's waiting for you."

"Thank you," I said numbly, as I steered Andrew towards the door.

There was something ominous about all this. As I opened the car door for Andrew, I felt it in the pit of my stomach.

When we arrived at Dr. Naidoo's office, he was outside in his garden, watering his plants.

"Hello, Andrew," he said, putting his arm around his shoulder. Then, shaking my hand, he asked, "Is your wife with you?"

"No," I replied.

"Please come inside," he said, as he took us through into his office.

I gave him the envelope. He took the CAT scan out and placed it on an illuminated screen on the wall. He pointed to a large, round, white shape on the negative image of Andrew's forehead.

"Mr. Luedi, I'm very sorry," he said gravely, "but Andrew has a brain tumor...it's here," he said, circumscribing the white area with his index finger, "in the left frontal lobe."

I felt my knees beginning to buckle. I reached for a nearby chair and sat down.

"How serious is it?" I asked weakly.

"Very serious," Dr. Naidoo answered. "You must fly to Sydney with Andrew tonight."

"That's impossible," I said, "there just isn't time to make the last flight."

"Well, first thing tomorrow then," he said as he picked up his phone and began dialing.

"I'm calling the Camperdown Children's Hospital to arrange for Andrew to be admitted there tomorrow for surgery."

****

By 8:30 a.m. the following day, Andrew, Marianne and I were flying south towards Sydney in a twin-engined Comanche—a plane owned and piloted by Alan Smith, a close friend of ours. I sat next to him with Andrew on my lap. Marianne sat behind us with Alan's wife, Lyn. Natasha was not with us. We had left her with friends.

The blue-green mountains and surf-washed beaches of Eastern Australia's mid north coast passed slowly beneath us. Untouched by their beauty, I sat there, staring ahead, tears rolling down my cheeks.

When we landed, our daughters, Claudia and Sandra, and a close friend, Rev. Kevin Sales, were there to meet us.

By noon that day, Andrew had been admitted to the Children's Hospital and accommodations had been arranged for Marianne and myself in the parents' quarters.

Later that day, as we sat at his bedside in a large ward containing about 18 children, the neurosurgeon's registrar came in to talk with us.

"Dr. Besser, the neurosurgeon who will be operating on Andrew, has discussed his case with me," he said, "The tumor is bigger than a baseball—about three or four inches in diameter. As well, there is a great deal of fluid. We'll have to reduce this before we can operate."

"When will that be?" I asked.

"Not for another week," he replied, "Monday, December 22nd. Dr. Besser will talk to you both tomorrow."

Dr. Besser was a quietly spoken man in his late 30s. As we sat in his office that Sunday afternoon, he emphasized the serious nature of Andrew's illness and went on to stress the urgent need for surgery.

"Unless we operate, Andrew will have only six weeks to live," he said.

"And if you operate?" I asked.

"Hopefully, this operation might prolong his life for a year, perhaps two years," he replied.

Marianne asked the question we were both thinking.

"Dr. Besser, what do you mean by *prolonging* Andrew's life?"

"Mrs. Luedi, he will be paralyzed and epileptic."

Upon hearing this reply, Marianne stood up and fled the office, weeping uncontrollably.

I stood there in confused and awkward embarrassment.

I could see in Dr. Besser's eyes an understanding of what Marianne and I were experiencing. There must have been numerous occasions when this dear man would have watched such heart-rending reactions to the solemn information he had to share. He quickly told me the other things I needed to know concerning Andrew's operation, so I could go without delay to comfort Marianne.

When I went to our room to do this, I realized that we both needed more than the comfort we could give each other. We had been emotionally shattered by Dr. Besser's prognosis and needed to find our strength in God.

I opened my Bible to Psalm 91. Together we read the opening words.

"He that dwelleth in the secret place of the most High shall abide under the shadow of the Almighty."

Marianne and I both knew that this was the only place where we could stand secure. As we read on, we began to sense that God would indeed give us His safety, His strength.

>> *"I will say of the LORD, he is my refuge and my fortress: my God; in him will I trust.*

>> *Surely he shall deliver thee from the snare of the fowler, and from the noisome pestilence.*

>> *He shall cover thee with his feathers, and under his wings shalt thou trust: his truth shall be thy shield and buckler.*

>> *Thou shalt not be afraid for the terror by night; nor for the arrow that flieth by day; Nor for the pestilence that walketh in darkness;*

nor for the destruction that wasteth at noonday" (Psalm 91: 2-6).

As much as I genuinely believed that God would sustain us through the trial we were about to face, I knew that I was presently so weak from the shock of it all, that I would not be able to survive it personally, much less, support Marianne.

This came home to me that very night, when, as Marianne and I were having dinner and I thought I was quite in control of myself, I suddenly broke down and began to cry.

I realized then, that, unless God did what He had promised to do in Psalm 91, neither of us would make it through this ordeal. So that evening, we went to the hospital chapel where we read and re-read this Psalm.

Next morning, shortly after I awoke, I began to go over again the terrible things that had occurred during these last few days. I began to pray and asked, "Lord, why did all this happen to us?"

Then the most extraordinary thing happened. In a split second, I saw in my mind a silver bar, the kind weight-lifters use to raise heavy weights. That bar was supporting a burden no human could lift. In the same moment, I heard in my mind the words, *'You should consider yourself privileged that I have chosen you!'*

Suddenly, my sadness was turned to joy. I wanted to sing. I also felt, inexplicable as it was, that Andrew would not die. From that moment, I experienced a strength and a buoyancy of spirit that I had never before known. From that point on, I did not shed another tear. I knew that God had given me His strength and that it would be enough to carry Marianne and myself through.

Since Andrew would not have his operation until the following week, I decided to make a quick trip back to Coffs Harbour to attend to the many things I had left undone because of my hasty departure. John Smith's wife, Faye, kindly agreed to come to Sydney to support Marianne while I was absent. During my brief visit to Coffs Harbour, I was surprised to discover that most of the community were aware of Andrew's illness and many wanted to help in some way. During these few days I was also able to make further arrangements for Natasha, who had been staying with friends, to come back to Sydney with me so she could see Andrew before his operation.

On the morning of the operation, Andrew was engaged in one of his favorite pastimes: drawing airplanes. As we both watched him finish this particular drawing, Marianne pointed to the bottom of it and said, "Andrew, put your name and the date down here, darling."

This disturbed me and I said to her, "Why ask him to do that, Marianne? Do you think this might be his last drawing—a kind of souvenir? Don't you have faith?"

Marianne pondered my words for a moment. Then, chastened by them, looked at me and said, "You're quite right...that was silly of me."

It was almost 8:00 a.m., the scheduled time for Andrew to be prepared for his operation. When a male nurse came by with a cart to pick him up, Andrew handed me his picture and said, "Dad, will you hang this up over my bed so I can see it when I come back?"

Marianne and I followed along as Andrew was wheeled into the elevator and up to the third floor. While he was being received there, by the team that would be involved in the operation, I noticed Dr. Besser. I went up to him. We shook hands. Then I said, "Dr. Besser, I'd like to ask you something."

"Yes, what is it?" he asked.

"Do you have children of your own?"

"Yes, I do," he answered. "And one of them is around Andrew's age."

I paused, unsure of how I could phrase my main question.

"Dr. Besser, if, when you are operating today, you feel that Andrew will end up seriously brain-damaged, will you...." I groped for the words, "...will you please let him die?"

My words, as I verbalized them, sounded callous, even brutal—not at all as I meant them to sound. I feared that Dr. Besser might even think I was in favor of mercy-killing, to which in fact, as a Bible believer, I am totally opposed. Yet as a pastor, involved for years with sick people, I was aware that it was now medically possible to bring a dying person back from the very brink of death, and then, although no quality of life was possible, to stave off clinical death almost indefinitely using sophisticated life-support systems.

Dr. Besser looked thoughtful, but did not respond to my question.

I then added, "There are a lot of people all over the world praying for Andrew."

"That may help," he answered, before moving off into the operating room.

We said good-bye to Andrew and they wheeled him away. We were not allowed to follow.

We knew that the operation would take five to six hours. It had been suggested that Marianne and I leave the hospital and return around 1:30 to 2:30 p.m.

We went to a nearby park where we both began to pray. Once again Marianne broke down and cried bitterly. This time I did not break down, nor did I cry. As I consoled her, I knew why God had given me a double portion of strength. In times of crisis like this, I realized I would have to carry Marianne as well.

At 1:30 p.m. we were back in the hospital waiting room. After 45 minutes, Dr. Besser came to us. He was still wearing his operating gown and cap, his face mask under his chin. He looked exhausted and his expression was grave.

"It was a very difficult operation," he said. "I'm afraid I couldn't remove the tumor. I succeeded in removing only one piece because there was so much bleeding...."

He put his hand to his brow and slowly shook his head—almost in disbelief. "It bled for hours—I just hope it doesn't start up again."

He was visibly upset as he added, "One thing is certain, it is a very primitive tumor. I suspect it is malignant, but to be certain I've done a biopsy and sent it to pathology. Andrew is in the recovery room now. You can go and see him."

We went in to see Andrew at once. In spite of the bad news we'd just heard, all we wanted to do was see our son. At least he had survived the operation. Our son was still alive.

He was coming out of the anesthesia when we went in. The upper part of his head was bandaged. Although he was pale and very drowsy, he recognized us. Then he said weakly, "I'm thirsty."

How relieved we were to hear him speak. And we were even more relieved when a senior nurse came in and he was able to answer her questions.

"Where do you live, Andrew?"

"Coffs Harbour," he answered.

"What color is your Dad's car?"

"White," he said without hesitation.

Marianne and I were delighted to hear these responses.

As soon as Andrew was back in the intensive care ward, Marianne went to phone our friends in Coffs Harbour.

I sat by Andrew's bed, holding his hand. Suddenly his grip tightened and he vomited. He leaned forward and vomited again. His whole body stiffened and he jerked backwards onto his pillow.

"Nurse! Nurse!" I shouted. "Come quickly!"

Andrew's eyes rolled back and he began to shake violently.

A nearby nurse, having heard my frantic cries, ran into the ward. Upon seeing what was happening, she rushed out again to get Dr. Besser, who was attending patients in the ward next door.

It was only a matter of seconds, before Dr. Besser was at Andrew's bedside. By this time Andrew, was lying motionless on his pillow— his mouth wide open.

Dr. Besser took his hand and tried to rouse him.

"Andrew! Andrew!" he called.

There was no response.

He pulled back the bed covers and, taking a silver instrument from his breast pocket, scraped it along the sole of Andrew's left foot.

"He's had a seizure," he said. "We'll have to operate again immediately.

"First we'll need a scan," he said to the nurse, "Organize it at once."

Even as he spoke, others on the staff began to appear. Each one responded instantly to his cryptic instructions.

As Andrew was being transferred from his bed to a cart, Marianne suddenly appeared, this time with Claudia and Sandra.

"What's happening?" she cried.

"Andrew's had a seizure," I answered. "They're going to operate again."

Marianne watched in horror, as the wardsmen and nurses wheeled Andrew out into the corridor, where they rushed him towards the elevator. She burst into tears. As Sandra and I tried to calm her, we saw Claudia disappearing down the corridor. With her background as a trainee nurse, she was anxious to get some medical information from the staff, who were trolleying Andrew away to radiology.

"Sandra," I said, "take Mum into the family waiting room and look after her there. I'll be with you shortly."

"Okay, Dad," she said, leading Marianne to the nearby stairway.

Suddenly I was alone.

I began to pace up and down along the silent corridor. With my fist clenched I began to pray. "Lord, I do not accept what I have just seen here, I stand against it. And I do not accept even the possibility that my son will die! You have given me assurance that your Scriptures are true, and I believe them. Psalm 91 speaks of your protection against the dangers and evils of this world. It speaks of life and not death."

"Because thou hast made the Lord, which is my refuge, even the most High, thy habitation; there shall no evil befall thee, neither shall any plague come nigh thy dwelling" (verses 9 and 10).

Then I began to recite in German the first few words of a hymn written by Martin Luther:

> *"Wenn Dein Wort nicht mehr soll gelten,*
> *Worauf soll mein Glaube ruhn?*
> (Should Thy Word cease to be true,
> On what foundation can I rest my faith?)"

"He will not die. Andrew will not die!" I kept repeating to myself as I went up the stairs to the family room.

Marianne was seated on a large sofa. She was still crying. Claudia sat on one side of her and Sandra on the other, trying unsuccessfully to pacify her. Also seated in the room were our pastor friend, Kevin Sales, and his wife. Everyone was silent and sober-faced. What a sad little assemblage it was.

I shook Kevin's hand. Then he said to me, "Marcus, we all have to face the fact that Andrew is not going to make it. It's now time for us to hand him over to the Lord."

"I refuse to accept that," I said stubbornly. "Andrew will not die. I believe he will come through this next operation. God will not let us down!"

There was a steely silence.

Then Claudia spoke.

"Dad," she said quietly, "I spoke to one of the doctors. He told me that Andrew's skull cavity was filling up with blood—like a balloon—and when I asked him what chance Andrew had of surviving, he said, 'Practically none.'"

Upon hearing these words, Marianne broke down again and began to sob loudly.

Claudia's eyes pleaded with me to be reasonable—to accept the medical truth of the situation. But her information did nothing to change my position. I began to quote Psalm 91 again. Andrew would live.

More silence.

"All right," said Kevin, "Let us all have that faith."

"But what if he dies?" Marianne burst out.

"He will *not* die!" I said.

Room 105

Chapter 19

Dr. Besser began this second operation at about 4:00 that afternoon. Andrew once again was on the operating table for almost five hours.

At 9:00 p.m. Dr. Besser asked to see us.

"Mr. and Mrs. Luedi," he said, choosing his words carefully, "Andrew has had a massive brain hemorrhage. I need to explain to you that the tumor, when I first operated this morning, was very vascular, that is; full of blood vessels, soft and jelly-like—very difficult to remove. However, this time, the blood in the tumor had clotted, and curiously this made the tumor more compact—so that I was able to remove a great deal of it.

"At this stage, I don't know how much damage has been done to Andrew's brain in the course of the operation. We've had to paralyze him totally to make sure he doesn't move and cause the bleeding to start again. If that were to happen there would be no hope. He is in intensive care on life support right now and there are tubes everywhere.

"I think before you go and see him, you need to be prepared by one of our senior nurses."

My heart reached out to this gentle-mannered surgeon. He'd been continuously on his feet since 8:00 a.m. that day. And for 10 of those 13 hours he'd been involved in the most delicate and demanding surgical procedures imaginable. And here he was now, on the point of utter exhaustion, doing all he could to ensure that we would not experience any further emotional suffering.

This had been a terrible day for our family. It was nevertheless only one such day for us. But for Dr. Besser, our black Monday was just another 'normal' work day and quite possibly only the first of several such days he would experience later that same week.

I reached out and gripped his hand tightly.

"Dr. Besser," I said, my voice charged with emotion, "I want to thank you for all you've done for us today."

After the nurse had told us what to expect, we went in to see Andrew. His head was heavily bandaged. There were tubes to the top of his head, into his arm, and also his leg. He was absolutely still. The only sound was the repetitious 'sssssss—phut—sssssss—phut' of the life support machine.

There was a hand-written note attached to the bed above his head. It read:

'THE PATIENT MAY HEAR AND FEEL
PLEASE TOUCH AND TALK TO HIM!'

We stayed with him until midnight, telling him over and over that we loved him, and also praying that God would take care of him.

When we returned to our room, we lay on our beds fully clothed, wondering whenever we heard the phone in the corridor, or footsteps on the stairs, whether it was bad news for us. Neither of us slept at all.

The next morning I went to see Andrew. Marianne lacked the courage to come with me. There appeared to be no change. However the resident doctor told me that Andrew had almost died during the night, but was presently holding his own.

I went back to Marianne and told her that he was still alive.

We spent the entire day beside Andrew's bed, again talking to him, touching him, and praying. There was no response of any kind. By evening, we could not help but wonder whether he would ever respond. Would he ever open his eyes? Would he ever talk or move again? Had our son been irreversibly brain-damaged, as I feared he might be? These and many other questions echoed and re-echoed through our tired minds. It was too much for Marianne. Once again she broke down.

The next day was Christmas Day. When I arrived to see Andrew early that morning, I was told that he had already been taken off life support and was now breathing unaided. How relieved I was. I went back at once to get Marianne. How wonderful it was, as we sat by his bed, just to watch his little chest rising and falling as he breathed—and we thanked God for it. It was an hour or more before we saw any other movement. When it came, we were both thrilled by it.

"Look, darling," said Marianne excitedly, "I think he's moving his fingers."

She was right. The fingers of Andrew's left hand were bending, ever so slightly, but bending nonetheless—a certain indication that he was not paralyzed, at least in his upper body and arms.

A little later he began to move his toes. It was as though our son was slowly coming back to us.

Later that morning we saw a tiny movement in his eyelids, then slowly he opened his eyes. For Marianne and me this was more wonderful than watching the most glorious sunrise. But there was, as yet, no recognition in those blue eyes of his—no indication that his brain was registering any visual impressions. There was nothing to suggest that he could hear anything either. However, early that afternoon, as we continued praying and talking to him, I noticed a tiny tear welling up in the corner of his right eye. Was he really responding to us at last?

"Andrew," I said, "give me a smile."

Almost imperceptibly we saw the corner of his mouth move, then curve upwards into a tiny, crooked smile.

Marianne and I were overjoyed. For both of us, this was the most wonderful Christmas present we had ever received!

Two days later, December 27th, Andrew was given another CAT scan. The results gave us further cause to be encouraged.

"I have some more good news for you, Mr. and Mrs.Luedi," Dr. Besser said to us, "The scan shows that Andrew is doing well at present. I am particularly pleased that he doesn't need a shunt to remove any further fluid from his brain."

That very morning, Marianne and I had been reading in Psalm

65, verse 8, how God is able to make both the dawning and closing of the day to rejoice. We had called on God to do that for us, and we believed He was already answering our prayer.

Dr. Besser was nevertheless only cautiously optimistic.

"The pathology report," he said, "indicates that Andrew's brain tumor is a particularly rare one. It is known as a central neuro-blas-toma. There are only 10 cases known in the world. Andrew is now the 11th."

"Furthermore, Andrew is the first person to have survived an operation to remove such a tumor," he added. "We are making medical history."

However, he went on to add that it was far too early for anyone to make a promising prognosis.

Later that afternoon, I received a phone call from *The Advocate* newspaper in Coffs Harbour. The information I gave them about Andrew's illness, its treatment, and our response, was published that night in a large front-page article with the headlines 'MIRACLE CURE FOR BOY, 7.'

Andrew remained in intensive care for the rest of the month. Although his ability to move physically was minimal during this time, he continued to make very gradual improvement. He was able to take solid foods but had to be fed by us. Although we constantly spoke to him, he never spoke a word—until the morning of December 31.

And what astonishing words they were. Nothing could have prepared us for what our son was to say to us.

Andrew was asleep when we arrived that morning. As we usually did, Marianne and I sat together at his bedside and held his hand.

When he began to stir, we spoke quietly to him.

"Good morning darling," Marianne said softly as she stroked his hand.

"Hi, Andrew," I said.

In an instant he was totally awake. His blue eyes opened wide and seemed to shine. There was no sign of his usual drowsiness as he looked hard at us, his mouth working as though he wanted to speak.

Then to our utter astonishment, he gasped in an urgent voiceless whisper, "I saw...I saw...angels!"

"You saw angels?" I asked.

"I saw...angels," he repeated with a conviction that indicated he was describing something he had actually witnessed—something as real as anything one might see in one's normal conscious state. This was not like the waking remembrance of some child's dream. Nor was it like the hallucinatory ramblings of someone who'd been on drugs.

I resolved to question him further.

"What did these angels look like, Andrew?"

My question seemed to excite him and again he tried to mouth the words before he could utter them.

"...Too...too beautiful!" he gasped.

"Did the angels say anything?" I asked.

"We love...we love...you!" he replied, his little face radiant as he said it.

Whatever had prompted Andrew's ecstatic words had also evoked a kind of emotional response we had never seen in him before.

But for Marianne and me, there was more to it than this. It was as though, in the midst of his physical weakness, our son had suddenly been revitalized—lifted up and borne along by some unseen power.

Could it possibly have been that the Lord, to Whom we had so fervently prayed, had actually sent His angels to do this as we had read in Psalm 91, verse 11?

"For he shall give his angels charge over thee, to keep thee in all thy ways."

This possibility was later to be confirmed in Andrew's life by evidence that even the most hardened skeptic would find difficult to disregard.

This angel episode had occurred on New Year's Eve, the very last day of 1986—the most difficult year Marianne and I had ever experienced. It was our hope that 1987 would be better. We prayed that, regardless of what this new year had in store for us, the Lord would give us the courage and strength we needed to meet its challenges.

Andrew came out of intensive care on New Year's Day. But he had to stay in the hospital for another two months. His terrible hemorrhage and brain trauma had taken away his ability to control his bodily functions, to feed himself and move his body and limbs in a coordinated manner. He was like a baby, who didn't even know how to crawl, and needed to be taught all over again how to do this, as well as all the other things children learn as infants. This involved an extensive physiotherapy program. Exhausting as it was for those of us involved, we were encouraged as Andrew began gradually to make progress.

This period of slow improvement was not without its setbacks. Barely a month after his operation, Andrew developed a massive blood clot in his right leg. It extended along a major artery from his ankle to his groin. The doctors treating him had never before seen anything like it in a child. The situation posed an awful dilemma. This life-threatening clot was able to be dissolved only by giving Andrew an anti-coagulant which, unfortunately, could easily cause his barely-healed brain to start bleeding again.

We had no other alternative but to give our permission for this to be done, even though we knew it could result in Andrew's death.

So, once more, we found ourselves praying, against great medical odds, that our son would survive. And once more the Lord was faithful. For when part of this enormous clot did, in fact, break up and go into Andrew's lung, as we feared it might, Andrew somehow survived. And when the recently-healed wound in his brain did, in fact, begin to bleed, he survived that too.

How we thanked the Lord, for preserving the life of our son, and for sustaining us, too.

It saddened us to see other parents who were suffering as we were, but, because they were not Christian believers, were trying to cope without the spiritual resources we had. We saw their frustration, their anger, and their despair. We longed to see them trust Christ as Savior and Lord, that they might know the peace and strength He brings in times of trial.

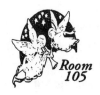

Chapter 20

O ne day in January, a young family came into the hospital with their five-year-old daughter. She was a strikingly beautiful little girl with glossy-black hair and dancing, dark-brown eyes. Like Andrew and all the others in the ward, she too had a brain tumor. Her bed was right next to Andrew's.

I asked the family where they were from and they said Korea. In a little while, they were joined by a few others, probably relatives and friends, we thought. Lying open on the little girl's bed was a large book on which oriental symbols were written.

"What kind of book is that?" Marianne whispered.

"I don't know," I answered. "The majority of Koreans are Buddhists. It could be a book of Buddhist writings—some sort of sacred text."

Some more Korean people came into the ward. When there were about nine or 10 of them gathered around the bed, one of the men in the group said something to them all in Korean and everyone knelt down. The man then began to pray—again in Korean.

"I'd love to know what he's saying," whispered Marianne.

As soon as he'd finished, the others prayed. This continued for about 30 minutes.

They had not long finished when our pastor friend, Kevin Sales, came into the ward to visit Andrew. How surprised we were to see that before he reached Andrew's bed, several of the Koreans went to him and shook his hand, greeting him by name and engaging him in animated conversation.

When he eventually arrived at Andrew's bed, I said to him, "Kevin, how did you come to know these people?"

"They belong to the Korean Christian Fellowship," he replied. "They hold their services in the same church building where my church meets in Lakemba. They are strong Bible believers and have come here to pray for this little girl, Ji-Hye, the only child of the Lee family from Seoul. Let me introduce you."

Then, turning to the group around Ji-Hye's bed, he said, "I want you all to meet Pastor Luedi and his wife, Marianne. And this is their son, Andrew."

The mention of Andrew's name sent a ripple of excitement throughout the group. Then the man, who had led their little prayer meeting, said, "Is this the Andrew for whom we have all been praying?"

There was soon a strong bond between our two families. Ji-Hye's mother, Soon-Chul, was a Christian, but her husband, Soo Guen, was not. He was still a Buddhist. When I suggested that they might like us to pray with them, they both readily agreed. They told us that a date had been set for Ji-Hye's operation and that Dr. Besser would be performing it. We told them how glad we were that they should have such a fine neurosurgeon and shared with them how wonderful he had been to Andrew.

The day before Ji-Hye's operation, her parents told me that a well-known Korean evangelist and faith healer would be at Sydney Airport, for a couple of hours that night, before flying on to Melbourne. They wanted to take Ji-Hye to meet this man, so he could pray for her healing. However, the senior nurse in charge of the ward told her that, now her daughter had been admitted as a patient due for surgery, this would not be permissible. They decided, however, that one of them should go to this evangelist and ask him to pray for their little girl's healing anyway.

The next morning, when Ji-Hye's operation was to be done, I was sitting by Andrew's bed. It was about 9:00 a.m. when the senior nurse came to see me. Marianne and I had got to know her very well during the time Andrew had been in the hospital. She appeared to be upset.

"Marcus," she said, "I need your help."

"Why, what's the problem?" I asked.

"As you know, Ji-Hye's operation is to begin in about two hours—and, believe it or not, her parents just told me that they don't want her to have it now! They flatly refused to sign the consent forms and when I tried to make them reconsider their decision, they walked out of my office into the corridor. I've no idea why they canceled out. Do you know what might have made them change their minds so suddenly?"

"I can't be certain," I said, "but it might have something to do with a meeting they arranged with a Korean faith healer."

"Marcus, as you well know, Ji-Hye is a very sick little girl," she said, "and she urgently needs that operation." Then, glancing down at her watch, she added, "Dr. Besser will shortly arrive to do it. I thought that since you seem to be friends with the parents, you might be willing to talk to them—get them to see reason. Would you do that Marcus?"

"I'll do what I can," I replied.

"Fine," she said, "come with me!"

She led me through the ward and then, via her office, into the corridor. Ji-Hye's parents were still there. But to my surprise, they were surrounded by seven or eight men, none of whom I'd seen before. They were all Koreans and all well dressed in suits and ties. Several of them were talking in Korean to Ji-Hye's parents, who looked very perplexed, I thought. Although I could not understand what was being said, I gained the distinct impression that these men were putting both parents under some sort of pressure.

As soon as I got their attention, I went up to the parents and, ignoring the others, spoke directly to them.

"I've just been told that you don't want Dr. Besser to go ahead with the operation," I said.

They made no reply.

"Can you tell me why?" I asked.

Soon-Chul glanced at her husband. Neither of them spoke.

Everyone was now silent as I stood there, with the senior nurse just behind me, waiting for some response.

When it came, it was from one of the Korean gentlemen. In very fluent English and, with a quite commanding presence, he said, "There is no need for the operation now. Last night several of us prayed that Ji-Hye would be completely healed. So you see," he said with a confident smile, "her tumor is gone."

"This is why," he added, "there is no need for Ji-Hye to undergo such a long and dangerous operation. It is quite unnecessary and pointless now, you understand?"

Ji-Hye

I most certainly did not understand, and was not about to say that I did.

"How can you be so sure that God has miraculously removed that tumor?" I asked.

"We who have prayed, know by faith that God has answered our prayers. For those who doubt what God has done," he went on with a condescending smile, "a brain scan will soon reveal that there is no longer any tumor."

I saw in this comment the only opportunity afforded so far to get this runaway train back on the rails. Turning to the senior nurse behind me, her head now bowed and a hand covering her eyes, I asked, "Nurse, could we arrange to have a brain scan?"

"I very much doubt it," she said brusquely. "There would not be time to do it before the operation. And in any case, a brain scan was taken only a day or two ago and it is perfectly clear, from what it showed, that she has a tumor."

As a highly experienced medical professional, she had been angered by what she had heard. This became increasingly apparent as she continued. "And furthermore," she said, addressing the parents, "if that tumor is not surgically removed—and soon—your daughter will die."

At that moment Dr. Besser came through the door at the end of the corridor. As he walked towards his office, the nurse went to meet him. The moment they disappeared, the Korean man who'd done most of the talking before, began once more to lecture both Soon-Chul and her husband, Soo Guen. I had little doubt that he would be branding the nurse, myself, and everyone else who thought the tumor might still be there, as faithless unbelievers. I was also pretty certain that he would be explaining away the fact that the last scan showed a tumor, only because it was taken before he and his friends prayed.

Poor Soon-Chul and Soo Guen; as I well knew from our own experience with Andrew, the strain of coping with a child's potentially fatal illness was stressful enough, without all this. I felt I had to try and help them.

"Could I speak to you privately for a minute?" I asked them.

I took them along the corridor, away from the others.

"I know exactly how you both feel," I told them. "And I want to say, that like both of you, my wife and I longed to see our child healed. And we too prayed, with others, that God would do it. But God, for reasons we do not understand, chose not to heal our son miraculously."

"But our friends say the tumor is gone now," said Soon-Chul.

I chose my words with the utmost care. "If God has healed your daughter, then that will be wonderful. But if, in His great wisdom, He has not done so, then, without an operation, she will die. I've an idea that might help you. Why don't you let Dr. Besser go ahead with the operation he's planned for Ji-Hye? If, when he opens her up, he discovers her tumor is gone, then he will close her up again—and you will have her back in less than an hour. But if, on the other hand, the tumor is still there, then Dr. Besser will remove it.

"What do you think?" I asked.

After a brief consultation with his wife, Soo Guen said, "Okay, we do the operation."

I went to the nurse and told her that they were now willing to go ahead as planned.

****

That afternoon, their little daughter emerged from the operating room with no sign of a brain tumor. Dr. Besser had successfully removed it in a five-hour operation.

That night, Soo Guen came to see me. In his broken English he said, "Marcus, I do not want to be Buddhist any more. I want to be Christian. And I have a question. Would you be my older brother?"

Room 105

Chapter 21

Andrew's progress was slow and laborious. Marianne and I became part of an intensive rehabilitation program provided by the hospital. This involved daily physiotherapy, speech therapy, and numerous other activities which we would need to continue, after Andrew was able to go home.

How grateful we were that the Boyce family, who had come to assist us at *Bethany* ministry, filled in for me during our stay in Sydney.

The program was psychologically and physically draining, not only for Andrew, but also for Marianne and me, as we prayerfully watched each day for the smallest sign of improvement and thanked the Lord whenever it occurred.

After many weeks of all this, I noticed that Marianne was becoming increasingly tired. I assumed that the unrelieved stress of Andrew's illness, operation, and now his two month recuperation, had brought her to a state of near exhaustion. My concern for her health deepened, when she began to experience severe pain in her shoulder and neck.

I suggested that she take some time off, from Andrew's program to rest up, but she would not hear of it. However, when the pain worsened, I insisted she have it checked out by the hospital doctors. They suspected she had pleurisy and treated her for this.

Around this time, I received a phone call from Bill in Coffs Harbour. He told me he had a buyer for the nursery. I was rather relieved to hear this. Indeed, the prospect of having both the nursery and Bill removed from our *Bethany* ministry pleased me greatly. I told Bill that, subject to certain conditions being met, I was in agreement with the idea of selling. He said he would negotiate a sale as soon as possible.

On February 18, 1987, some 10 weeks after Andrew's second operation, Dr. Besser decided that he was well enough to go home.

When our plane landed at Coffs Harbour, we were greeted, not only by a large group of friends, but also by the press. Andrew's illness and remarkable recovery had been widely reported and his return home was headline news.

So when our frail, spindly-legged little boy emerged from the plane, he was greeted by cheering and applause. He came slowly down the steps, then, to our astonishment, walked falteringly, but unaided, across the tarmac and into the arms of his waiting friends. He was a celebrity.

God had mercifully preserved the life of our son. How long that life would continue, we did not know. But Marianne and I firmly believed that, as we faced this next challenge, we would be given the wisdom and strength to do all that would now be required of us.

As soon as media interest had subsided, we began to make plans for this next phase of our lives. I realized that, because of my heavy involvement in the *Bethany* ministry, most of the onerous responsibility for Andrew and his rehabilitation would fall upon Marianne. Whilst I was grateful for the many Christian friends who offered their help, I knew that coping with Andrew would still be a full-time job. And, in addition to this and the ongoing household responsibilities, there were the needs of our youngest daughter, Natasha, who was only 12 years of age and needed time with her mother as she entered her adolescent years.

It would be taxing for all of us, but particularly so for Marianne.

The greater part of our married life had involved us in a succession of severe difficulties and hardships—all of which Marianne had borne without complaint or regret. I wondered how many wives would have coped, as cheerfully and resourcefully, with living in the places where we had lived since arriving in Australia. I thought of the very basic accommodations on Jack's Woolgoolga property—its lack of amenities, especially its hillside privy. I remembered as well how we had all lived cheek-by-jowl in the trailer parked next to our first commercial garden. And then of course those stressful years of ministry, first in the inner-city parsonage at Newtown and then the succession of mainly temporary country dwellings here in the Coffs Harbour area. I recalled not only the sheer physical difficulties of these years, but also the psychological and spiritual challenges they had brought.

And on top of all this, the most harrowing time of all—that of Andrew's illness. This had taken a heavy toll on all of us—especially Marianne.

Inwardly, I shrank from the prospect of having her, without any respite, move into this next phase with all its stresses.

However, Marianne was adamant, as I expected she would be. She saw this as just one more battle we had to fight and that we would fight it exactly as we'd fought all the others—in the strength of the Lord on the basis of Philippians 4:13. *"I can do all things through Christ which strengtheneth me."* So we asked the Lord to enlighten and strengthen us, then prayerfully worked out what we would need to do, and began to do it.

For the next two months, while I attended to the ministry, Marianne took responsibility for Andrew's medication and rehabilitation program. Andrew responded well and, over this period, we saw slow but steady improvement in his ability to speak and control his physical movement. After some six months, it was decided that he might soon be ready to spend a short session each day at school. This began in early July. Marianne sat with him in class on each of these occasions. I did this too as often as I could.

Before becoming ill, Andrew's language ability, especially his reading, had been quite outstanding and fortunately his radical brain surgery did not seem to have diminished it. In fact, he still read better than most of his classmates. However, his mathematics skills were quite another matter. He had lost his numerical ability completely and had to be re-taught the most rudimentary concepts and operations.

In general however, Andrew did commendably and eventually was able to become a full-time pupil again. Although he still had a long way to go, Andrew had made remarkable progress academically.

But perhaps even more remarkable, was the progress evident in his character. Whereas earlier, he had been a typically self-focused seven-year-old, he now began to show unusual concern for the welfare of others. For example, one day when he was at the swimming pool for his hydro-therapy, a lady in a wheelchair was wheeled by. He watched her, with rapt attention, as she was being attended to and asked, "That lady, is she all right?" Even when assured that she was, his obvious concern for her continued and he repeated his question.

Andrew's compassionate attitude toward others was seen often in his insistence upon others being given preference over himself and this aroused comment from several who observed it.

Along with his love and concern for others, his interest in spiritual things grew apace. This was evident in his disarming enthusiasm about his Savior and Friend, the Lord Jesus Christ. Whereas before his illness he was reticent even to mention His name, now he referred constantly to Jesus Christ and his love for Him. Repeatedly, he would ask me to tell him about the birth of Christ and share with him a range of Bible stories about Him. Frequently, he would tell others of his encounter with the angels.

Andrew was a changed boy.

On April 25, a thanksgiving service was held in the Coffs Harbour Baptist Church. It was packed with people, most of whom had prayed for Andrew when he was so sick. Many came long distances to be at this special service. Among them were Ji-Hye and her parents. Ji-Hye had made a good recovery and Andrew was thrilled to see her again. He said that he would marry her one day!

Room 105

Chapter 22

It was shortly after this when I noticed that Marianne was finding it difficult to cope with Andrew's rehabilitation program. Although the Boyces, and others, were helping her as much as they could, I could tell that she was not managing effectively. Each evening, when I came back to the house, she was close to exhaustion. I noticed, as well, an unhealthy puffiness in her face and body. When she began to experience severe pain around her lungs, I arranged for her to have a thorough medical check-up.

As occurred when she had shoulder pain in Sydney, nothing sinister was revealed and she was prescribed tablets which, it was hoped, would help her. Unhappily, this treatment brought no significant improvement and she continued to lose ground physically. I noticed also that she was becoming emotionally depressed because Andrew, in spite of all the assistance he was receiving, was not yet coping as well as she had hoped he would. Although Marianne was deeply disappointed by this, it did not deter her from continuing to throw herself into his educational program, almost with abandon. Her commitment to the medical aspect of his rehabilitation was just as zealous. She was determined that Andrew would do *all* his exercises and get *all* his medication, in spite of her failing health.

One day, when I came home, I found her sitting silently in our living room. The curtains were drawn and she held her head in her hands.

I sat down next to her on the arm of her chair.

"What's the problem, darling?" I asked gently, putting my arm around her shoulder.

She did not reply. Her eyes were closed. I brushed her hair back and kissed her lightly on the forehead.

She opened her eyes and looked blankly ahead. "Marcus...I'm so tired," she sighed. "I don't know what's wrong with me."

Then, turning her head towards me and pleading with her eyes, she said, "Darling, I'm so tired...you've got to take over Andrew's program...I simply cannot do it anymore. You'll have to do it."

I saw something in her eyes that had never been there before. It was defeat. My dear wife, who had been such a source of strength to all of us for so many years, had finally reached the limit of her human strength and resolve—and was now telling me so.

"Of course I'll look after Andrew for you," I reassured her.

Then she said something I did not expect. "Marcus, I want you to know everything about Andrew's program, especially his medication—the whole regime—because, when I'm not here, it will be your job to look after Andrew."

Marianne was saying, as clearly as she could, that she was going to die, and was taking the necessary steps to prepare me for it and to set things in order.

"Marianne, please don't talk like that. You are not going to die. I'll certainly take over Andrew's program because you are not well. But you will not die!" I protested.

"Marcus," she said, taking both my hands in hers, "hear me out...there's something more I want to say. You must marry again. Andrew needs a mother."

"Marianne, don't talk of death," I chided. "Do not even think about dying. I'll take care of Andrew until God makes you well again."

Over the next few weeks I took care of Andrew as I promised I would, but Marianne's health did not improve. In fact, it deteriorated. Her pain intensified and fluid began to accumulate between her heart and lungs.

Further tests failed once more to reveal the cause of her illness. The accumulation of fluid, in her pleural cavity, made it difficult for her to breathe and it was decided to aspirate it with a large needle.

This process was excruciatingly painful and had to be repeated at regular intervals. By mid-October I had become so concerned about Marianne's condition that I arranged for her to be flown, by air-ambulance, to Sydney for specialist attention in Royal Prince Alfred Hospital.

Because I had to take care of Andrew and the *Bethany* ministry, it was not possible for me to accompany her. However our dear friends, John and Faye Smith, offered to go down to Sydney to be with her while she was in the hospital there.

Marianne was admitted on the morning of Monday, October 31, 1987. That evening I phoned her.

"How are you, darling?" I inquired.

"Fine," she responded. "I had some tests today."

"Did they find anything?"

"They said they needed to run more tests to discover what's really causing the problem."

"When will they be doing that?" I asked.

"Tomorrow," she answered. "How's Andrew, darling?"

"Okay."

"John and Faye have been marvelous," she added.

"Please thank them for me."

"They're both right here. You can speak to them yourself if you like. Here's John."

I phoned again the next day. Once more Marianne told me that they were running additional tests to identify the underlying problem. This battery of tests continued every day of that week, as I discovered from my nightly phone calls to her.

By Friday, I was concerned that there was still no firm diagnosis.

When I phoned that evening, the tone of Marianne's voice was somehow different—rather subdued.

"Marcus, you'd better pray—seriously—I've been told that I have only three months to live. I have terminal cancer."

"Are they sure it's cancer?" I asked.

"There's no doubt about it. It's right through my body. The pain I had in my shoulder, back in January, was caused by cancer eating into my bones."

"When did you find this out?"

"On the day I arrived—Monday."

"But you told me on Monday that they were going to run more tests."

"Yes, they were—because they wanted to find the primary site of the cancer and they still haven't located it."

"But why didn't you tell me all this on Monday?" I asked with a note of anger that I regretted, immediately after I heard myself.

"I just couldn't tell you...I didn't want to hurt you," she replied.

"Darling," I said, "I suspected you had cancer—even expected it. Knowing this for certain now doesn't hurt me...because I *know* that God will heal and restore you, as He did Andrew."

Silence.

"This is just another challenge we'll have to face—as a family. God's name will be glorified when you are healed."

"I hope so," Marianne said.

As soon as I put down the phone, I decided to break this news to the girls.

I began by calling Claudia in Sydney.

"I already know, Dad," she said. "Mum told me on Wednesday, when I went to see her in the hospital down here. I told Sandra too."

"Dad," she continued, "why has God allowed this to happen to Mum—especially after all we've been through with Andrew?"

"Claudia, I am certain that God's purpose is to heal Mum of cancer, so that the miracle will bring glory to Him. I have no doubt about it. He did it with Andrew and He'll do it with Mum. You believe that, don't you, Claudia?"

"Yes I do, Dad."

When I spoke to Sandra, I got a similar response. But I wondered how Natasha, the youngest of our daughters, would react.

I told her what the doctors had said, then went on quickly to assure her that her mother would nonetheless be healed and that God would be our strength at this dark time. I quoted the first two verses of Psalm 46, Scriptures which Marianne and I had both claimed, just before she was flown to Sydney.

"God is our refuge and strength, a very present help in trouble. Therefore we will not fear, though the earth be removed and though the mountains be carried into the midst of the sea" (Psalm 46:1,2).

Also, as confirmation of my conviction that God would raise Marianne up, I quoted; "*The Lord will preserve him and keep him alive*" (Psalm 41:2).

"So you see, Natasha," I added, "although the doctors say that Mum has terminal cancer, we have God's Word that, like Andrew, she will not die. We mustn't worry."

"I'm not worried, Dad," she assured me. "I believe Mum will be okay."

I then took Andrew aside and simply told him that his mum would be in the hospital for a while longer and then would be coming home. I arranged for the Boyces to look after Natasha and Andrew and keep an eye on *Bethany* ministry, so that I could fly to Sydney and be with Marianne.

When I saw her, she was unexpectedly bright and in good spirits. The doctor in charge of her case told me that she had a very positive attitude and that this would help her significantly to cope with her illness.

I sat by Marianne's bed and told her what I had shared with the girls—namely that God would raise her up, in spite of the medical diagnosis. Once more, I read Psalm 46 to her, then showed her the parts of Psalm 41 I believed gave confirmation that God would do this. I drew her attention, in particular, to verse three, which tells how David, the Psalm writer, was languishing on a bed of sickness. Then I went to verse eight, which referred to an "evil disease" which, it said, "cleaveth fast unto him."

I read this verse in a modern translation (NIV) where the nature of David's illness was depicted as terminal. "*A vile disease has beset him. He will never get up from the place where he lies.*" I explained to Marianne how, in the verse before this one, David's enemies (who were faithless unbelievers) had imagined the worst for him and so had said there was no hope of his surviving.

I likened this situation to the one we were now experiencing, where doctors, who lacked the faith we had, had given us a hopeless prognosis. Then I read verse 10 from the same modern translation.

"*But you Lord have mercy on me; raise me up that I may repay them.*"

"Marianne," I said, as I gripped her hand, "the Lord will raise you up to confound all those who doubt that He can and will heal you."

While Marianne and I were talking, Ji-Hye's parents, and some other Koreans who had heard of Marianne's sickness, arrived. I read these passages to them also. They too took them as confirmation that Marianne would be made well.

They were all the more encouraged in this belief because, like us, they had a little child who had been a cancer victim, and, by the grace of God, was still alive and doing well.

Later that day, the doctors on Marianne's case recommended that she be given a course of chemotherapy immediately.

After discussing it with Marianne, I gave them permission to do this the next day. On her 47th birthday, Marianne underwent her first treatment of chemotherapy—a double dose.

It made her violently ill. I was so distressed by her reaction, that I went to the doctor in charge. "Is this treatment really necessary?" I asked. "Will it help her?"

"Mr. Luedi, we cannot cure your wife's cancer. We are giving her chemotherapy in an effort to prolong her life."

"But Doctor, this is making her so terribly ill and distressed. She doesn't want to have any more."

"Unfortunately, some patients react in this way."

"Well," I said, "if it can't cure her, and it only makes her desperately ill and miserable, I fail to see what positive purpose it serves. She's gone through enough already. I'd like you to stop it—and we'll leave Marianne in God's hands."

"I can't say I blame you, Mr. Luedi," he replied.

The chemotherapy was discontinued and within a few days Marianne and I came back to Coffs Harbour.

This homecoming, unlike Andrew's earlier that year, was a sad one. Our return became even more unhappy when we found that Bill, while I'd been in Sydney with Marianne, had sold the nursery and absconded with all the proceeds. The purchaser was a 50-year-old woman called Colleen. Shortly after our return, she came to me and said, "Marcus, would you please come and look at the plants in my exotic section?"

She led me into the greenhouse where there were large numbers of elkhorns, staghorns, orchids and other protected plants.

"Look," she said in dismay, as she fingered the withering brown leaf of a giant staghorn, "they're dying."

I could see she was right.

"I assume you've been watering them regularly?" I said, as I examined a couple of others more closely.

"Yes, I have—daily," she replied, looking over my shoulder. "What could I have done wrong?"

"Probably nothing," I said. "These plants all smell of kerosene. Someone has poisoned them."

"Who on earth would want to do that?"

I did not answer as I continued to inspect more plants, most of which smelled of kerosene. When I turned around, she was staring at me in shocked disbelief, her hands to her mouth.

"Oh, my goodness...you don't think that he...Oh no!" she gasped, "...he wouldn't...would he, Marcus?"

I did not know how to respond to Colleen's question. I suspected that Bill might have done this as a vindictive act, but could not imagine his motive. So I simply said, "Colleen, none of these plants which are dying have a label to show that they have been legally acquired for commercial purposes. If someone had wanted to prevent their being used, as evidence in an official inquiry, he might decide to destroy them by dousing them with kerosene."

Colleen soon realized that her days as a nursery proprietor were numbered.

Within a month, *Potter's Nursery* bore a sign which said, 'CLOSING DOWN SALE'.

Bill's disappearance with the nursery money was financially ruinous for us. But what happened a few weeks later was even more disturbing, especially for poor Marianne.

Room 105

Chapter 23

O ne afternoon, when I came home from the farm, Marianne met me at the door. She was very agitated. She held a letter in her hand.

"Marcus," she said as she handed it to me, "the sheriff came here with this today."

It was an eviction notice from the bank which held the deeds of the property we were leasing for our *Bethany* ministry. It stated that the bank was foreclosing, because one of the property owners had failed to repay a loan of several hundred thousand dollars.

"Darling," she added, "it says we've got to be out of here nine days from now! And it says this is a *second* eviction notice. What's going on? Was there a *first* eviction notice?"

"Yes, there was," I answered. "It came when we were with Andrew at the hospital in Sydney."

"You didn't tell me about it."

"No, I didn't," I replied. "You had enough on your mind with Andrew. So I phoned one of the lessors up here in Coffs Harbour. He told me that the notice was a mistake—that the matter was being currently settled in court. He said it had nothing to do with us and that I should ignore it."

"Then why this notice?" Marianne asked.

"I don't know," I said, "but I'll find out. I'll phone the man I spoke with before."

When I contacted this man and told him we'd been served yet another eviction notice, he was very apologetic.

"Marcus," he asserted strongly, "the case was settled last week in court. I have no idea why you were sent that notice."

"But what should I do about it?" I queried.

"Ignore it," he replied. "I'm well aware of the terrible strain you are under right now—with both Andrew and your wife so sick. You don't need any more pressure. Look," he added, "to put your mind at rest, I'll arrange for you to phone our lawyer, who'll confirm what I've said."

I told him I was willing to accept his explanation and that a phone call to his lawyer would not be necessary.

Because Andrew had been under the spotlight of public scrutiny since his illness, it was not long before news began to spread throughout the district that now, his mother also had cancer.

When someone contracts such a serious disease, there is no lack of advice forthcoming from people who want to help. As Marianne's condition worsened, I received letters, phone calls and visits from those who were keen to tell me how she could be made well. Some recommended medical remedies which, they claimed, were 100% effective. Others, who knew we were Christians, urged us to adopt certain spiritual remedies.

And what a range of these there were. Some of them were quite bizarre.

For example, we received a handkerchief from someone who lived 3,000 miles away in Western Australia. Enclosed with it was a letter reminding me that, in the period of the early Christian Church, handkerchiefs which belonged to the apostles had the power to heal diseases. The letter assured us that the enclosed handkerchief had been properly prayed over and, if laid upon Marianne's body, would have the same miraculous effect. Remedies of this 'spiritual' sort came from a range of religious backgrounds.

For instance, an overbearing lay pastor, who was of an extreme Pentecostal persuasion, visited me often. On each occasion he would insist that I pray with him and that I claim total healing, while he interceded for me in tongues.

Then there was George, the ultra-conservative preacher, who

made a five-hour car journey from Brisbane to give me a 10- point list of things Marianne and I needed to repent of, before God would bestow healing.

"Cancer is of the devil," he avowed, "and by your disobedience, you have given ground to Satan. And that is why your wife is now dying of cancer."

Needless to say, I did not allow any of these strange people to come near Marianne.

Another man, an elderly gentleman, who was a former treasurer of the local Baptist Church, stopped me in the street one day and inquired after Marianne. I told him that although there had been a marked deterioration, I firmly believed that God would nonetheless raise her up.

He looked at me with searching but compassionate eyes, then gently said, "Marcus, I am praying for God's grace upon you and your family when Marianne dies."

As I always did, when someone spoke of Marianne's death, my immediate reaction was to reject his words. They brought me no comfort and in fact unsettled me.

As Marianne became progressively weaker, I tried my best to care for her. This responsibility, together with my commitment to Andrew, the *Bethany* ministry, and Natasha, began to weigh heavily upon me. I became particularly concerned about Natasha. I knew that without her mother, her crucial needs as a young teenager were not being adequately met. I, and many others, began to pray that the Lord would undertake particularly for Natasha and would also enable our little family to cohere during this demanding time.

I had been told in Sydney that Marianne would be gone by Christmas. Yet when Christmas came, she celebrated it with us in a small French restaurant at Nambucca Heads, south of Coffs Harbour. She survived into the New Year, but by mid-January, was in constant pain and on morphine. Her breathing became so labored that she had to be taken to Coffs Harbour Hospital and placed on oxygen.

She was back home again by February, but was now bedridden and required 24 hour care. This involved full medication and oxygen, both of which I administered every day. Somehow, by the grace of God, I continued to do this. Once again, I could not have managed without the support of the Boyces, who cooked our meals, helped me with Andrew and Natasha, and assisted with *Bethany*.

During this time, the boys involved in the commercial garden work and ministry would often come to our house to seek my help with urgent problems.

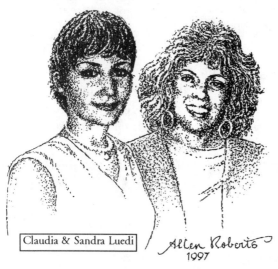

Claudia & Sandra Luedi

Allen Roberts
1997

When Dr. Scott, our family friend and physician, came on his day off to see Marianne and myself, he saw how hopelessly over-committed I was. He took me aside and said, "Marcus, this cannot go on. If you continue trying to do what I see you doing now, you'll have a nervous breakdown within a week. Marianne will have to go to a private hospital. There is no other alternative, I'm afraid."

That afternoon, an ambulance came to take Marianne to the hospital. I sat in the back with her. As we pulled out of our drive, I looked back through the rear window at our house and farm. As I did so, the thought crossed my mind that Marianne would never return to this place again.

The notion was repugnant to me and I immediately tried to banish it from my thoughts. "Marianne will be healed," I said to myself. "As sick as she is, the Lord will raise her up and will bring her back to us."

So that Marianne could have someone with her all the time, I organized a 24-hour roster of ladies who were willing to come when I could not.

Marianne had been in the hospital only a day or two when Dr. Scott invited me around for dinner. Following our meal we went into the living room where his wife, Jocelyn, served us coffee. After a few minutes of casual conversation, Dr. Scott looked at me and said, "Marcus, I need to tell you, that in my considered opinion, Marianne has only about three weeks to live."

I looked straight back at him and resolutely said, "Ian, from a medical point of view, what you say may well be true. But *I* believe that God will intervene and heal her."

I made this statement with all the conviction I could summon. But even as I spoke the words, the image of Marianne—her face thin and lined with pain—crowded into my mind. I knew, as one who had pastored many people who were terminally ill, that my wife had the appearance of someone who would soon die.

As I looked Dr. Scott in the eye, I tried to visualize Marianne as I longed for her to be—strong, healthy and cancer-free. I then did what I had been struggling to do continuously over the past few weeks. I called on God to make the image of Marianne, I had conjured in my mind, a reality.

Over the next two weeks, Marianne lost weight rapidly. Her face and body became emaciated. She could not breathe now without an oxygen mask and was given large amounts of morphine to reduce her terrible pain.

I visited her twice a day. When she was unable to talk, I would just hold her hand and pray, claiming from God the total restoration I kept imagining in my mind. When she was awake, I would read the Scriptures to her, constantly exhorting her to trust God to raise her up. When she was well enough, we would also discuss a number of the books we had read on the subject of divine healing. On these occasions, I would sometimes read to her the passages from those books which I had underlined as especially significant.

One day when the minister of Coffs Harbour Baptist Church was visiting Marianne, he beckoned me as he was leaving her room, and we both went outside. "Marcus, Marianne is very low," he said, "I think you should tell your daughters in Sydney to come and see their mother."

Clearly he was of the opinion that, if Claudia and Sandra did not come at once, they might never see their mother alive again. Whilst I did not share his opinion, I did not argue with him, but told him I would do as he suggested.

The following afternoon, Sandra arrived from Sydney. As I drove her to the hospital, I tried to prepare her for the shock I knew she would experience when she saw her mother.

"Mum has aged so much since you last saw her," I warned. "You'll barely recognize her."

When Sandra saw her mother, she was devastated. She burst into tears and ran crying from the room. I followed her at once and found her in the arms of a nurse who was trying to pacify her. As emotional as her reaction was, she regained her composure fairly quickly and said, "Dad, I want to go back in to Mum now. I'll be all right."

She went to the bedside and Marianne reached up weakly with open arms. They hugged for a few moments without speaking. Then Sandra said, "I'm sorry Mum."

"That's all right, darling," replied Marianne, "I understand. It's so good to see you."

Claudia arrived the following day. When she saw Marianne, I could tell that she, too, was shocked by her appearance, but tried hard not to show it. At about 7:00 that evening, it was time for me to go home to Andrew and Natasha. Claudia and I walked arm in arm along the corridor adjacent to Marianne's room. As we came by the ward desk, the nurse in charge there caught my attention, then asked, "Mr. Luedi, have you a moment, please?"

"Yes, of course," I replied, approaching her desk.

"Which funeral director have you chosen?"

I was totally unprepared for this question. I had been so pre-occupied with Marianne's healing that the matter of a funeral—much less a funeral director—hadn't even crossed my mind.

I didn't know what to say. Then I recalled the name of a man who had conducted some funerals for me when I was a Uniting Church pastor in the area.

"Er...Keith Logue," I mumbled. "He's a friend of mine."

The nurse wrote down this name and I walked with Claudia towards the entrance.

"They have to ask those questions," I whispered, as I put my arm around her shoulder. "I guess they just don't understand that Mum is not going to die."

As we stood by the entrance, I placed both my hands on her shoulders and said, "Let's keep believing that, Claudia. You do believe it, don't you, darling?"

She kissed me, then held me close. "Of course I do, Dad."

The nurse's question about a funeral director had threatened my belief that Marianne would be miraculously restored to health. I felt that I now needed to exercise my ailing faith to restore and strengthen my spiritual position again. So I went home and drafted an outline of the praise service that would be held when Marianne was healed.

My main concern was now Natasha. Although she had been with us since Marianne was hospitalized, she had steadfastly refused to visit her. Whenever I suggested that she come with me, she would say, "No, Dad, I don't want to see Mum while she is so sick. I'll wait until God has healed her."

Since I had constantly encouraged her in the belief that Marianne would be completely healed, there was really nothing I could say to this.

However, my concern for Natasha increased when, on the following Monday evening, she came to me and complained, "Dad I'm feeling dizzy."

I could see she was lonely.

The next morning she complained again of dizziness and I allowed her to stay home from school. Since her dizziness continued, due, we later found out, to an inner-ear infection, I kept her out of school for the rest of the week.

I became acutely aware that this little daughter of ours, who had never displayed her feelings publicly, was suffering inwardly. She desperately needed loving reassurance. In my present emotional state, I seriously doubted whether I could even begin to meet her needs.

On the Friday evening of that week, upon returning from the hospital, I said to her, "Natasha, you have not been to school for these last four days. Have you been getting dizzy because of Mum's illness?"

"No Dad," she replied emphatically. "I'm not worried in the slightest about Mum's illness. I know that Mum will be healed, as Andrew was."

The next morning, Saturday, March 12, 1988, at 5:20, the phone in my study rang.

It was a message from the hospital.

"Mr. Luedi, your wife has just passed away. I'm sorry."

Room 105

Chapter 24

Marianne's death shattered me.

Even after I'd seen her body at the hospital, I still found it impossible to accept that she was gone.

It was about 6:30 a.m. when I arrived back home. Everything was silent as I walked towards our front door.

I had no idea how I would break the news to my children.

Andrew, who was an early riser, was already up when I came into the entry hall.

"Hi, Daddy!" he cried, as he hugged me around the waist, "Where have you been?"

"Andrew," I said, "I've just been to the hospital. Mummy has died."

His reaction was quite extraordinary. His face lit up and, clenching his little hands gleefully, he shouted, "Mummy's in Heaven! Praise the Lord! Mummy's in Heaven!"

I wondered for a moment whether he had really comprehended what I'd just told him.

"Mummy has died," I repeated slowly.

"Mummy's in Heaven! Mummy's in Heaven!" he shouted again, this time jumping up and down and clapping his hands gleefully.

Suddenly he stood still. He frowned, then said thoughtfully, "Oh...that means I won't see her anymore." Then, after a pause, his face became quite radiant and he added, "But she's with Jesus now!"

I knelt down and hugged him.

"Yes, Andrew," I murmured, as much to myself as to him, "You're right. Mummy's with Jesus now."

I was certain, as I held him to me, that he did understand—perhaps better than any of us.

With some foreboding, I prepared myself to tell Natasha. When I entered the bedroom, she was curled up, on the bed there, as though still asleep. She turned her head towards me.

"Dad," she said flatly, "you look sad."

"I *am* sad darling," I responded quietly.

"Why?" she snapped angrily.

"Mum has passed away," I said as calmly as I could.

In the next instant, her face was contorted with anger.

"I know!" she shouted vehemently, throwing back the blankets. "I heard Andrew calling out and clapping his hands when you told him Mum had died—and I didn't want to believe it!"

She then went and got a bag, threw it on to her bed and unzipped it. Then wrenching open her cupboard door, she reached in and began to pluck items of clothing from hangers and drawers.

"I'm leaving this house now!" she fumed, stuffing each item into her bag. "I can't bear to look at Mum's pottery for a moment longer."

She zipped up the bag, threw her school uniform over one shoulder and grabbed her school things.

"Take me to Cherie's place—right now," she demanded as she pushed passed me. "Let me know when the funeral's on!"

I realized it would be futile to try and reason with her, so I drove her to her girlfriend's house.

On my return, I began making the many phone calls that were necessary. Claudia and Sandra were both now back in Sydney, so I phoned them first.

When I called Claudia and told her that Marianne had died, she did not say anything for several seconds. Her silence evidenced the fact that, like me, she too had been stunned by what had happened.

I was unable to make direct contact with Sandra, so asked a friend to pass on the message. Both Claudia and Sandra left Sydney by train that evening. I met them at Coffs Harbour Station early the next morning.

Although they were bearing up bravely, I could see that they had been severely shaken. Marianne's death had dashed the firm conviction that God would heal their mother.

As I was putting their baggage into the trunk of my car, Claudia said, "Dad, before you drive us home, would you please take me to see Mum's body?" I did as she asked and drove to the morgue at Keith Logue's funeral parlor. When we pulled up outside, I asked Sandra whether she wanted to come in with us.

She declined.

Claudia stood by the open casket, her eyes brimming with tears.

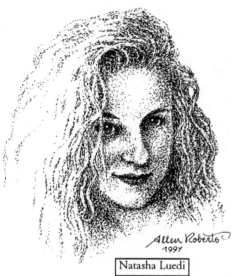

Allen Roberts
1997

Natasha Luedi

Then, with calm conviction, she said, "Now I believe that Mum really is gone."

She was bridging the gap between the lost hope of healing and the grim reality of death.

As I left the mortuary, with my arm around her, I realized that I, myself, had not yet even begun to come to terms with the loss of my wife and its faith-shattering implications.

We had been home for only a short time when I received a phone call from George, the man who had given me the 10-point list that he maintained would ensure Marianne's healing, if I met its demands.

"This is George," he said. "I've just heard the news. I'm sorry your wife is dead, but I knew it would happen. You didn't do the things I wrote down, did you? Right after I left that list with you, I went off and prayed. And I knew then—in my spirit—that you wouldn't repent and that your wife would die. Your wife's death could have been avoided. And it's all your fault!"

I was in no frame of mind to deal with this man. So I terminated his telephone tirade by gently laying my phone down on its handset.

Around noon that day, as I watched Claudia and Sandra preparing our midday meal, I realized that they, and my other two children, would be looking to me for support over these next few days—especially at the funeral. In my present state I knew I was incapable of doing this. I'd been stunned by Marianne's death and, because she had not been healed, had been asking God why ever since—and was getting no answers.

I'd come to the end of the road.

I was utterly defeated. I knew it. I accepted it.

Then, suddenly, I heard myself saying: "God, I have no idea why you took Marianne, but I accept it." With the uttering of these words, my deep disappointment with God was suddenly gone. In its place I sensed an infusion of strength and peace that I knew would sustain me.

I went immediately to my phone and called the minister who was planning to conduct the funeral service and said to him, "Graeme, you'll recall that, when you asked me yesterday if I would like to take part in the funeral service, I flatly refused. Well now I believe I can do it. I'd like to bring the eulogy tomorrow."

"Marcus," he replied, "I'm very pleased. I'll pray for you as you prepare yourself to do it."

A very large number of people attended that service. It was a blessed time when God met us in our grief, and we watched Him minister to everyone present. The Lord did indeed strengthen me to deliver the eulogy, in which I looked back on our 22 years of married life.

I recounted how God had led us through unusual circumstances to come to Australia, and I told how He had used Marianne to bring me back to Christ; an accomplishment for which she would surely receive a reward in Heaven. I said that Marianne was not only a good mother and a great companion to me, but that she also had a heart for the needy, the broken-hearted and the homeless.

The extreme Pentecostal man, who prayed in tongues for total healing, was notable by his absence. In fact he never spoke to me again and went out of his way to avoid me.

However, the elderly treasurer, who told me he would ask the Lord to bestow His grace when Marianne died, came up to me at the funeral and pressed into my hand an envelope containing $500 to help me meet the funeral expenses. This man's practical expression of help touched me deeply.

The funeral was over. The people who'd come with their words and embraces were now all gone—brief blossoms, bloomed and gone.

Each had his own life to live. Each his own hardships and sorrows to bear. Each his own loved ones to care for.

As one who had counseled the sick and bereaved, I knew that the loneliest time was to come; that life without Marianne, the wife and the mother, somehow had to be lived....

Room
105

Chapter 25

Natasha perhaps was hurting most of all. She refused to talk of her mother's death. She would not be consoled, even by those closest to her. She would lock herself in her room, refusing to speak to anyone. On one such occasion, Jean-Pierre tried to get her to open her door. When at last she did, and he tried to take her into his arms, she stiffened and grimaced and turned her head, rejecting him totally. It was to be years before she could bring herself to talk to him, or even look at him again

Claudia and Sandra both returned to Sydney. Andrew and Natasha both went back to school. Once more, I began to manage the *Bethany* ministry, whilst trying to be both father and mother to my two younger children. The Boyces, and other thoughtful Christian friends, helped out wherever they could.

Letters poured in, most of them encouraging, though a few of them not so. One of the latter came from a Christian lady. In it she wrote: "What kind of God is it who would heal the son and take away the mother?"

I had found it personally necessary to lay aside such why questions; but now this woman's words had opened up an unhealed wound. I still had no answer to her query. But I knew that questions of this sort could easily lead one to impugn the character of God. This, I would not allow myself to do. Having determined instead, on the day before the funeral, to trust God, without asking such loaded why questions, I disregarded her letter.

The central issue for me at this time, was not why God had led me through these pathways of suffering, but whether He was a God who could be trusted. Martin Luther, in one of his quotations, strongly asserted that He was trustworthy:

> "I don't know the way He guides me.
> But well do I know my Guide!"

These words, along with others from the Bible, enabled me to face each new day. The words of Romans 8:28 were lifelines for me: *"all things work together for good to them that love God, to them who are called according to his purpose."*

Another passage from the New Testament enabled me to see that, no matter how severe the pruning, I could trust in God as a caring gardener, Whose aim was to bring forth fruit. *"I am the true vine, and my Father is the husbandman. Every branch in me that beareth not fruit, he purgeth it, that it may bring forth more fruit"* (John 15:1,2).

In the months that followed, although I was not fully functional as a Christian, I knew that in spite of all my unanswered questions, the God Whom I had *unquestioningly* trusted was graciously sustaining me, day by day.

During this time, I took a far less active role in the church. There were two reasons for this. The first, was that I wanted to devote more time to my children and to *Bethany*. The second, was that I was not yet ready to take up again the kind of preaching ministry I had exercised before. I felt I was totally unqualified to exhort believers to call on the Lord to supply all their needs in Christ Jesus. Furthermore, whenever I heard anyone preaching on the subject of faith, I felt as though a sword had pierced me through. Such messages did not move me to exercise my own faith at all. Indeed, to my shame, I found myself asking, "What does he know about faith? I exercised more of it than anyone!"

I began to realize then that I was still blaming God for not healing my wife when He had encouraged me to believe so strongly that He would. I was still feeling that He'd let me down—and not only me, but my children too. I had encouraged them all to believe what I believed. And because they had not reached my faith position for themselves, they had, in a sense, fed on my faith—only to be spiritually disillusioned and damaged, as I had been, when Marianne died. I knew that many others who had looked on me, as a man of faith, had also crashed with me at that time.

What had gone wrong?

Had God made a mistake?

Of course not, I reasoned. He is perfect. The mistake cannot be His.

Then could it have been my mistake? I failed to see how. God's mind is revealed in His Word—the Scriptures. And I had claimed and even visualized Marianne's healing, on the sole basis of what God had said.

I knew that to be a genuine man of faith, who was of any use to God or man, I would have to resolve this issue—and soon. So I prayed that the Lord would show me how to do it.

My prayer was answered sooner than I expected, through a man whom the Lord brought across my path.

That man was Oscar Hauser, one of my own countrymen. Oscar was an elderly pastor from the Evangelical Brotherhood Church in Switzerland. Curiously, he had known me there in my early youth and had just arrived in Coffs Harbour to replace another pastor who was on a 12-month furlough.

I took the opportunity, shortly after he arrived, to visit him and his wife. Oscar was a mature, wise man, and I felt confident about sharing with him this problem I'd been praying about.

As we sat together in his study, I told him that, when Marianne was so ill, I had found certain Bible verses which I had claimed as promises from God that Marianne would be healed. I told him how, I'd then sought and found, other Scriptures (or rhemas as those in the healing movement often called them) which confirmed this. I also showed him how I had used what Dr. Paul Yonggi Cho, in his book *The Fourth Dimension* called 'guided visualization' whenever I prayed, actually imagining my wife as I longed to see her—in the full bloom of health.[1]

Without interruption, Oscar heard me out.

"I think I might have a book here which could help you, Marcus," he said, as he ran a finger along the volumes on his bookshelves.

He located a paperback, took it out, and began to flip through its pages.

"There's a particular part here...that I think you will find interesting," he mused, as he opened the book, then turned it around and handed it to me. "Page 33, the second paragraph."

I began to read. It was about the Korean evangelist and healer, Dr Paul Yonggi Cho. It succinctly summed up the teaching of his book, *The Fourth Dimension*; an important part of this teaching being that "God had created the world through the power of his 'imagination' and that man as a 'fourth dimension' spirit being can also create his own world through the power of his imagination."

I knew from my own reading of Yonggi Cho's works, that this was truly what he taught. Indeed, I had not only read it, but firmly believed it.

I read on into the following paragraph, where reference was made to the prayer technique of "visualization," which I had actually practiced when I asked God to heal Marianne.

It seemed to me, however, as I read this section, that those who had written this book I now held in my hand, were not in favor of visualization. In fact, they were warning that this very technique was the one used by occultists.

On the same page they had stated, categorically, that this 'visualization' and 'imagination' procedure was the basic one used by sorcerers.

What I was reading was beginning to disturb me.

What's this book about, I asked myself, *and who wrote it?*

I glanced at the front cover and saw that it was titled *The Seduction of Christianity: Spiritual Discernment in the Last Days.*[2] It was co-authored by Dave Hunt and T. A. McMahon. I was not familiar with either of these writers.

I then turned to the back cover, where I read: "The Bible clearly states that a great Apostasy must occur before Christ's second coming. Today Christians are being deceived by a new world view more subtle and more seductive than anything the world has ever experienced."[3]

Having read this, I paused. I knew that the Bible warned believers not to be deceived by false teachers and false prophets. And I was particularly aware that in the gospel of Matthew, chapter 24 verse 11,

Jesus Christ Himself had said that false prophets would arise—especially in the last days prior to His return.

Could this guided visualization, of which I was so strong an advocate, be part of such a deception?

Surely not! As a Christian believer, how could I be deceived? Yet I had to admit that the Lord Jesus Christ, in speaking of the signs and wonders performed by false prophets, warned as well, that, *"if it were possible they shall deceive the very elect"* (Matthew 24:24).

My eyes skipped down to the final two sentences on the back cover. As I read them, my anxiety increased.

> "The Seduction of Christianity will not appear as a frontal assault or oppression of our religious beliefs. Instead, it will come as the latest 'fashionable philosophies' offering to make us happier, healthier, better educated, even more spiritual.
>
> "A compelling look at the times we live in. A clear call to every believer to choose between the original and the counterfeit. Only then can we hope to escape THE SEDUCTION OF CHRISTIANITY."[4]

I looked up at Oscar. He was standing there, in front of his bookshelf, his blue eyes—highly magnified behind powerful lenses—holding me in their patient, kindly gaze.

I had been psychologically and spiritually shaken by what I'd just read.

"Oscar," I said grimly, "if what this book suggests is true, then I've been terribly deceived. Yonggi Cho has been my mentor. His book has been a kind of prayer handbook for me as I've prayed for Marianne's healing."

"Why don't you take this book home with you and read it right through?" Oscar suggested.

I did so. I found it to be a carefully and well written book. Within a couple of days I'd finished it. I was deeply challenged. The book began by showing that every Christian should be aware of the danger of being despoiled by the empty deception of counterfeit worldly philosophies. To support this from Scripture, the writers made reference to something the apostle Paul wrote to the Colossian believers:

"Beware lest any man spoil you through philosophy and vain deceit, after the tradition of men, after the rudiments of the world, and not after Christ" (Colossians 2:8).

The authors then pointed out that, although these counterfeits might have the appearance of being scriptural, they are not. They gave a wide range of evidence to show that many teachings on how to achieve things through prayer, were, in fact, based upon well-established occult practices.

The book carefully examined the healing movement. Many of its widely accepted practices were convincingly shown to be part of an age-old tradition of pagan shamanism or sorcery, brilliantly disguised as Christian. It showed as well that those purveying these teachings often used the Scriptures deceptively, to give their teachings a biblical veneer.

The well-documented chapter on this subject began with another quotation from the apostle Paul, indicating that a time would come when believers would not even desire sound teaching:

"For a time will come when they will not endure sound doctrine, but after their own lusts shall they heap to themselves teachers having itching ears; And shall turn away their ears from the truth, and,shall be turned unto fables" (2 Timothy 4: 3,4).

As I read all this, I began to realize that my longing to see Marianne healed had made me unusually vulnerable to false teaching. The more I read, the more I realized that the authors, Hunt and McMahon, were working from a solid basis of Scripture to reveal what was the true and what was the counterfeit. As a Bible-believer, this encouraged me.

I was further encouraged by the fact that these counterfeit teachings, which they were lining up against Scripture, had been carefully researched and properly documented.

I was particularly impressed by the balance and tone of the book. It showed not only what was *wrong* about the beliefs and practices it examined, but what was *right* according to the Word of God.

As soon as I'd finished the book, I phoned Oscar and told him I needed to see him as soon as possible.

He probably detected the anxiety in my voice and invited me to come across to his house right away.

"I've read the book," I said, as I went with him into his study.

"What did you think of it?" he asked, as we sat down together.

"Oscar, I am convinced that what it says is true. I need to repent. I now see clearly that I have embraced the teachings of man rather than the Word of God. And I also see that these teachings—which I've not only believed, but put into practice and recommended to others—really do have their roots in occultism.

"And, Oscar," I went on, "all four of the writers whose teachings I applied and recommended, are listed in *this* book you gave me: Yonggi Cho, Agnes Sanford, Francis McNutt and Richard Forster—they're all here—every one of them!" I said, jabbing the book with my forefinger.

"Oscar," I said with shame, "I studied most of these authors and shared their philosophies on healing with Marianne to encourage her, when we knew she had cancer. She read many of them for herself. Agnes Sanford's book, *The Healing Light*,[5] particularly impressed her. She read it constantly during her final stay in the hospital—it lay on the table next to her bed the day she died.

"Brother," I said with anguish and regret, "I really do need to repent of what I've done!"

We both bowed our heads.

I asked the Lord to forgive me for believing and embracing manmade doctrines and allowing them to overrule—and even replace—His Word. I renounced them and asked Him to enable me to turn from them, rejecting every false teaching I had imbibed and trusting only the Scriptures as my authority. I also asked for His grace to put right those things I had said and done which had misled and hurt others—especially those of my own family. I thanked the Lord for working through Oscar, and the book he'd passed on to me, to show me the error of my position and establish me in His truth.

As I opened my eyes, I said, "I need to speak to Claudia, Sandra and Natasha right away."

At the earliest opportunity I did this. I tried to explain to each of them, that although the Lord *had* raised Andrew up and preserved him to this day, this did *not* provide me with a warrant to claim—or virtually demand—Marianne's healing, as I'd done. I told them that I now realized that God does not grant healing because of some "prayer formula," or because of some "rhema" confirmation we may think we have in Scripture. I told each of them that I had taken unbiblical teachings on board, and on this basis, had misled them into believing that their mother would undoubtedly be healed.

I also went to others who had stood with me on the basis of my unscriptural healing position. I told them, too, that I'd been wrong.

As I embarked upon this path, I realized that my erroneous beliefs on healing had been communicated far beyond my family and friends. I had begun sharing these beliefs publicly before Marianne became sick. The nature of my position on healing had been widely reported in the press when Andrew was so ill. As I recalled some of the things I had been quoted as saying, I was embarrassed, and all the more so because of my attitude as I had shared them. My comment on Andrew's early recovery was published widely in a number of Australian daily newspapers. One of these typical quotes was:

"'I'm feeling strong now because the promise is for full recovery and we will not accept anything less,' Marcus said yesterday." [6]

To some, these might well have been words of great faith. But I now saw them as an expression of unwarranted belief about healing that was close to presumption, even arrogance.

I did not feel this way because my wife's death had weakened my faith. In point of fact, my faith was stronger now than it had previously been. For, having realized that I had been beguiled into depositing my faith in mere men and their beliefs, I was now resolved to put it where it really belonged—in the God of the Bible.

As far as Andrew was concerned, I had come to understand that he had been healed, not because I had claimed that God had to do it in response to something I had discovered in Scriptures or elsewhere to make Him do it. God is not obliged to do what we want. He will not be badgered. He had healed Andrew because, in His own infinite wisdom, He willed it for His own purposes. He had a purpose, which none of us could really know, for prolonging Andrew's life. So He did it, and Andrew was still alive. But this was no warrant for me to believe He would necessarily preserve Marianne's life.

I did not know or fully understand why God did not heal

Marianne. But I did know that had she been healed, I, in my doctrinally confused state, would have erroneously attributed it to the unscriptural prayer techniques I employed to secure her recovery. And, in addition to this, had she recovered, this would have confirmed for me (and perhaps for others) that the teachings on healing which had ensnared me were not false, but of God.

As I thought upon this, I knew that had Marianne been healed, nothing would have held me back from testifying to the authenticity of the counterfeit I had adopted. I would very probably have joined the ranks of those leading the healing movement and exercised a full-time ministry to teach and practice healing world-wide.

Whilst I knew that I could never hope to take back or correct all the things I had said publicly, I felt I should at least try to put things right in the churches where I had spoken on healing. So I made arrangements to do this by speaking to several church congregations in the Coffs Harbour area. On each of these occasions, I explained how and why I'd gotten off track in this matter of healing. I pointed out, that I had been subtly influenced by dubious teachings to take a position that, on the surface, appeared to be scriptural, but in reality was not. To illustrate how a minor change in one's doctrinal position can lead to major consequences, I quoted a striking illustration I'd recently come across in Dr. Francis Schaeffer's book *The Great Evangelical Disaster*.

> "Not far from where we live in Switzerland is a high ridge of rock with a valley on both sides. One time I was there when there was snow on the ground along that ridge. The snow was lying there unbroken, a seeming unity. However, that unity was an illusion, for it lay along a great divide; it lay along a watershed. One portion of the snow when it melted, would flow into one valley. The snow which lay close beside would flow into another valley when it melted.
>
> "Now it just so happens on that particular ridge, that the melting snow which flows down one side of that ridge goes down into a valley, into a small river, and then down into the Rhine River. The Rhine then

flows on through Germany and the water ends up in the cold waters of the North Sea. The water from the snow that started out so close along the watershed on the other side of the ridge, when this snow melts, drops off sharply down the ridge into the Rhone valley. This water flows into Lake Geneva—and then goes down below that into the Rhone River which flows through France and into the warm waters of the Mediterranean.

"The snow lies along that watershed, unbroken, as a seeming unity. But when it melts, where it ends in its destinations is literally a thousand miles apart. That is a watershed. That is what a watershed is. A watershed divides. A clear line can be drawn between what seems at first to be the same or at least very close, but in reality ends in very different situations. In a watershed there is a line." [7]

I explained to the believers with whom I shared this illustration, that I had allowed myself to be persuaded, to stand doctrinally on the wrong side of God's line—with disastrous results. I also explained that Christians today were on a critically important watershed which concerned the nature of biblical inspiration and authority.

Having read *The Seduction of Christianity* [8] and gone back to the Scriptures in respect of this whole healing matter, it seemed as though a veil had been lifted from my eyes. And when I'd told those I'd misled that I had been wrong, it was as though a mounting burden had tumbled down off my back.

I had been brought by the Lord as a pupil into His school in the valley of suffering and sickness. And here, I had begun to learn that in this matter of healing—as in every other aspect of the Christian life—it is, and ever must be, as the Lord Jesus Christ acknowledged to His Father in the depths of His anguish at Gethsemene,

"O my Father, if it be possible, let this cup pass from me: nevertheless not as I will but as thou wilt" (Matthew 26:39).

Room 105

Chapter 26

For the next few months, life began to return to normal, or so it seemed, until the day I returned home and found an official letter attached to my front door.

To my astonishment I found it was a third and final notice of eviction. A copy had been sent to every person living on the property. It ordered us to vacate the premises within nine days.

I realized in horror that I had been misinformed by the lessors when they advised me to ignore the earlier notices. I phoned the bank from which the notice had come and told them everything that had happened. However, their course was firmly set. They were foreclosing and said that if we, and everything we owned, were not out of the place within those nine days, they would have us forcibly removed.

We all knew that it would be impossible to vacate the property within so short a time. Since the local branch of our bank refused to extend this period, I decided to go over their heads to management level in Sydney. I wrote a two-page letter which described, in detail, the circumstances leading to the current situation and faxed it off at once. Within 24 hours I was told (by a representative of the bank corporation management) that we had been granted an extension of time, sufficient to enable us to vacate the premises and sell as much as we could at such short notice.

With the vacating of our property and the hasty sale of all our assets, the *Bethany* Ministry came to a close.

In the last 12 months I had lost my wife to cancer. I had almost lost my son to cancer, and he was now handicapped. I had lost all my money, my home, and now my ministry. In spite of all this, I knew that the Lord was still with me and was working through His pruning and molding process for His own good purposes. However, the stress of all this upon me was soon to take its toll.

About two weeks after we had vacated the premises, I was driving through the main street of Coffs Harbour, when I suddenly felt a kind of shock jump from the top of my head across to my left shoulder. It was as though electrodes had been attached to me and then a high voltage current had been turned on.

I immediately became dizzy and feared I would lose consciousness. I thought I might be about to have a heart attack, or perhaps a stroke. So I pulled in at once to the curb. After a minute or so, these symptoms subsided. But when I stepped out of the car, they began again. I went straight to my doctor, Ian Scott, and he referred me at once to a Coffs Harbour cardiologist, Dr. Ross Walker, whom I also knew personally.

Dr. Walker gave me a thorough examination which included some stress tests. While he was monitoring me on his treadmill, I began to black out. He grabbed me before I collapsed and helped me to a chair. When I had recovered, he sat down and began to talk to me.

"Marcus, I am well aware of the terrible stress you've gone through. You're in poor shape and your children need you," he said. With these comments he went to his desk and began to write a letter. "I'm referring you to a specialist in Sydney. He'll arrange to see you later this week. I'm asking him to do an angiogram which should tell us whether you have a heart problem."

Even as I left the office, the symptoms returned. They continued, on and off, for the next few days.

As I sat in the departure lounge of the Coffs Harbour Airport, I looked out through the glass doors of the terminal building at the runway.

Memories began to flood back—memories of the many times I had brought Andrew and Marianne to and from aircraft out there on that tarmac, when they were so desperately ill.

And now it was I who was ill.

Dr. Walker's comment came back to me. "...Your children need you."

It triggered off other thoughts, doubts and nebulous fears—fears of what might happen if, this time, *I* were the one who was incurably ill. And my two dependent children—what would happen to them?

I could feel the stress mounting, as these thoughts surged back and forth inside my mind. My head began to swim. The electric current leapt again from my head to my shoulder. My neck and arm muscles tightened. They were almost in spasm. I waited, my head in my hands, for the inevitable blackout.

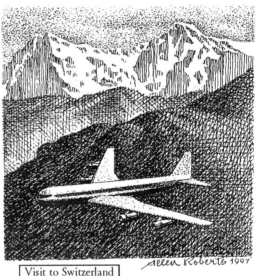

Visit to Switzerland

It came, as I feared it would. After it had passed. I wondered whether I would be able to make the trip to Sydney. *If I had a heart condition*, I thought, *I might not even survive long enough to get to the hospital there.*

I knew I was starting to panic, but could do nothing to stop it.

I felt so wretched, I thought I might die—right there and then.

Almost involuntarily, I took out my pen and notebook. I began to scribble in it the rough draft of a will—outlining instructions concerning the apportioning of my few meager possessions to my children. I continued writing, even though I knew I was out of control and that what I was doing was ridiculous.

When it was time to board my plane, I quickly stuffed the notebook and pen into my pocket, took my boarding pass and joined the queue at the terminal door.

The angiogram and various tests they ran in Sydney showed that there was nothing wrong with my heart, and as far as they could ascertain, I had no other serious physical illness.

However, the specialist who examined me said that I was physically and psychologically exhausted. In his opinion, the acute stress I had suffered, had brought me to the point where a nervous breakdown was imminent.

He advised me, as a matter of urgency, somehow to organize my life so that I could go away and recuperate.

On my return to Coffs Harbour, arrangements were made for me to do this. The Boyces once more offered to look after Andrew for me. The parents of Cherie, Natasha's friend, agreed to have her stay in their home during my absence.

I had no idea where I would go until I received a letter from my brother, Gideon, in Switzerland. In it, he offered to pay my air fare to Switzerland and the United States, so I could unwind and spend time with my relatives and also those of Marianne.

I left Australia on October 2, 1988. I was overseas for six weeks and during this period was able, for the first time in many years, to have a holiday. There was time to relax, in the company of relatives and old friends in both Europe and America; time to share with them what had happened to us all in Australia, and when, on my return journey I spent a week completely alone in Hawaii, time at last to weep.

Room 105

Chapter 27

On my return, because I had no home to go to, I lived with Natasha and Andrew in a trailer. Later, we moved into rented accommodations. I was just able to manage financially, because of a single-parent pension, for which I was now eligible. Fortunately, I was able to supplement this by growing and marketing exotic fruit, while Andrew and Natasha were at school each day.

This simple and uncomplicated arrangement enabled me to devote more time to my children than I had ever been able to do before.

In the following year, 1989, Dr. Besser gave Andrew an encouraging report in which he wrote that there was no evidence of any recurrent tumor. In the year after that, Andrew was taken off all medication. The removal of this responsibility was a great help to us all. It made it easier for his teachers at school, as well as for us at home. It also lessened the burden of those dear folks who cared for Andrew when he spent his week at Camp Quality—an international organization established to provide enjoyable camping activities for terminally ill children.

Both of the children were doing well at school, Andrew in the fifth grade of elementary school and Natasha in the 11th grade of high school.

I was especially pleased to see how Natasha, without any prompting from me, had slipped unobtrusively into the maternal role to help meet Andrew's needs. When her little brother needed new clothes, she would go shopping with him. When his hair needed cutting, she would do it. She was determined that he would be well dressed, though rather more trendily than I'd have done.

In October 1991, it was time for Andrew's final medical check in Sydney. The night before, I gave him the special tablets one is required to take before having a brain scan, and put him to bed.

At 4:30 a.m. I was suddenly awakened by a curious noise. It came from Andrew's room. It was a sort of quivering staccato groan. I rushed in to find Andrew in the throes of violent convulsions, foaming at the mouth and vomiting. I wondered whether it might have been caused by the brain scan tablets, but Dr. Ian Scott discounted this when I reported what had happened. What Andrew had suffered, he said, was an epileptic seizure.

I was most upset to learn this. Andrew had been doing so well up to this time; and without warning, we had to contend with the fact that the poor little lad was now epileptic. I remembered, all too well, the terrible seizure he'd had in the Camperdown Children's Hospital five years ago, just before Dr. Besser had operated on his giant tumor. I was unnerved by the possibility that this seizure could have been caused by the regrowth of that tumor.

Dr. Besser, when he examined Andrew's brain scan later that day in Sydney, thought not. He could find no indication of a tumor, or anything else that could have triggered off this latest problem. He thought it might have been caused by the heavy scarring associated with Andrew's earlier brain surgery. He prescribed tablets, which he hoped, would control the epilepsy.

These, and other tablets, were effective in staving off further seizures for the next five weeks or so. Then, towards the end of this period, something happened which caused us further alarm. He began having severe bouts of vomiting and, as these persisted, he started to lose weight. Dr. Naidoo arranged for him to be sent, by air ambulance, to Sydney and admitted to Camperdown Children's Hospital, where we had spent so much time before.

For Andrew, this hospital had been like a second home. He settled in quickly. Some of the nurses, who looked after him before, were still there and they greeted him like an old friend. He told me that he enjoyed being in the hospital. When I asked him why, he said, with a grin, "Because the nurses love me so much!"

The place was not so pleasant for me. The whole familiar scene evoked a kind of déjà vu experience. Its blood tests, scans and EEGs made me feel as though I was stepping onto the same medical merry-go-round which had whirled us about just five years ago.

These tests took about three weeks. During this time, Andrew, as usual, began to make many new friends. One of them, Glenn Smith, who was recovering from a brain tumor, became a special companion. Glenn's parents, John and Rhonda, took a particular interest in Andrew and I became friends with them too.

The tests, that had been run, revealed no sign of cancer or anything else of a serious nature. So Andrew was discharged the day after Christmas. However, he continued to lose weight, which concerned me greatly. Dr. Gaskin, a gastroenterologist who saw Andrew at the Sydney hospital, shared my concern when he saw him in February of that year (1992). He told me that he thought Andrew's trouble was neurological—probably caused, as I had feared, by a tumor.

Andrew's pattern of weight loss and vomiting continued throughout the ensuing month. In less than six months he had lost 14 pounds, a great deal of weight for a little boy of his size. Although he was looking forward to attending Camp Quality again, he was just too ill to go. This was unfortunate, since these camps, with their wonderful programs, had become the highlight of Andrew's year. He loved the friendship of the other children and had responded particularly well to his adult companion, one of whom was always assigned to each child. A deep and lasting bond had been established between Andrew and Nicola, a young Coffs Harbour medical student, who was his companion on his first camp, just after Marianne's death.

Dr. Naidoo, like Dr. Gaskin in Sydney, also suspected that Andrew's problem was neurological and insisted that he be re-admitted to the Children's Hospital, so that his illness could be accurately diagnosed and treated. This was done just prior to Easter, 1992, and further exhaustive tests revealed in fact that there was a tumor—this time in the brain stem, where breathing, speech and other vital functions, are controlled. The tumor was only the size of a pea but, because of its location, was almost inoperable.

I discussed the options we now had with Dr. Besser.

"Mr. Luedi," he said, "having carefully examined Andrew's scans and x-rays, I would say that an operation would be very complicated and dangerous—far more so, even, than the ones I performed some years ago."

"What are Andrew's chances of successfully coming through such an operation?" I asked.

"He'd have no more than a 50/50 chance I'm afraid. If I were to do it, I would insist that he regain at least four pounds in weight."

Dr. Besser could see that I was indecisive.

"Perhaps you'd like some time to make up your mind," he added. "Come and see me when you've done that."

I decided to tell Andrew that he had another tumor and that Dr. Besser might have to operate again to remove it. When I'd related all this to him, Andrew was thoughtful. Then after a few moments he asked, "Why do I have another tumor, Dad?"

"I don't know, Andrew," I replied, "Only God knows why."

He appeared to be unperturbed by the situation, which he knew was causing me such concern, and simply said, "Dad, I love God. And Heaven is my home."

Later that day the Registrar, a young woman in her mid-twenties, came to me and said, "Mr. Luedi, I understand you are considering an operation for your son, Andrew—and that if you decide to go ahead with it, you'll have Dr. Besser do it."

"That's so," I replied.

"Let me say to you, that Dr. Besser is probably the only surgeon in Sydney who could tackle such a difficult and risky operation. I thought you would be encouraged to know this."

The next morning I went to Dr. Besser and told him I would like him to operate. What option did I really have? I thought that if Dr. Besser could indeed remove the tumor, then Andrew mightn't need any radiation or chemotherapy. After all, the little fellow responded well after his first operation. And, honestly, in view of the circumstances, I didn't have the physical strength to go through all that again. I left it with God and the doctor's advice.

Dr. Besser set aside a day in June and I returned with Andrew to Coffs Harbour, where he was admitted at once to the local hospital and tube-fed to regain his weight.

Although confined to bed with a tube in his nose for two weeks, Andrew never complained and spoke often, to those who attended him, of his love for the Lord.

One day, the Chief Medical Administrator said to me, "Mr. Luedi, what a wonderful boy your little Andrew is. We often discuss him in our medical staff meetings. He gives us so much and we are all enriched by having him here."

On Friday, June 1, Andrew was back at the Children's Hospital.

Early that morning, before he was taken to the operating room, I washed his hair and prayed with him, exactly as Marianne and I had done five years ago.

****

It was almost noon when Dr Besser came into the waiting room and asked me to come with him into his office.

"How is he?" I asked anxiously.

"He's okay," Dr. Besser said, "but I'm afraid I couldn't remove the tumor. All I could do was remove a sample for biopsy. It is obviously the same tumor he had before. I tried three times to remove it, but whenever I touched it, his blood pressure dropped. If I'd persisted, I'd have had a dead boy on my hands. Mr. Luedi, I'm so sorry that this is all I've been able to do. You'll be able to see Andrew in the recovery room quite soon."

I thanked Dr. Besser for all he'd done, then went into the waiting room next to the recovery ward. My friend, the Reverend Kevin Sales, who had supported Marianne and me when Andrew was operated on before, was there once more to encourage me.

After a few minutes, a nurse called us into the recovery room.

Andrew, his head heavily bandaged, was just about to regain consciousness. He opened his eyes and, recognizing me almost at once, raised his right hand and made a "V" sign with two fingers.

"Victory in Jesus," he said.

Room
105

Chapter 28

Within the next week, Andrew was out of recovery and into the neurological ward, where he was prepared for his first five days of chemotherapy. With him, in that ward, was a 10-year-old girl called Lisa Augustine. Like Andrew, she too had a tumor in her brain stem which could not be surgically removed.

While they were both having chemotherapy, I got to meet Lisa's parents, Steele and Joanna. Whenever they came to see their daughter, they were dressed immaculately, he in a formal business suit and she wearing fashion clothing and jewelry. I guessed they were both involved in a prosperous business venture of some kind. They subsequently told me they were in real estate, both here and overseas.

The total course of chemotherapy, prescribed for both Andrew and Lisa, was to continue for at least 12 months. The process was long, complicated, and tedious. For Andrew it included first another operation which involved a central-line that would enable cancer-shrinking substances to be continuously infused intravenously. There were as well, of course, the necessary daily blood tests and other monitoring procedures.

For most of each day, Andrew lay in bed with tubes attached to his nose and body. The chemotherapy caused unpleasant side effects such as fatigue, nausea, high temperature, infections and, after a few weeks, hair loss. Andrew experienced all of these, but as usual never complained.

As I sat with him each day, I sometimes could not help but wonder whether all this was really worthwhile. The parents' information sheet gave no guarantees. It stated that although chemotherapy may be of benefit in prolonging a child's life, the tumor is likely to come back.

As I looked at Andrew and his friend, Lisa, who lay in the bed next to him, I had to accept the hard truth that this treatment was really only a temporary measure at best. However, my present attitude, toward Andrew and his illness, was completely different to the one I'd had when Marianne was dying.

On that occasion, I would not come to terms with the real medical situation. I was in denial. But now, by God's grace, I was able to face and accept that Andrew was indeed terminally ill.

When Marianne was so ill, I was claiming, even demanding, that God heal her. But with Andrew, I now had handed over the whole situation to the Lord and was trusting Him to have His way, regardless of the outcome.

With Marianne, I had been continually in turmoil and under stress, as I longed for the outcome that *I wanted*, but that the Lord was not willing to give. But with Andrew, I genuinely desired only God's perfect will and was at peace. This time, I really understood what Spafford, the hymn writer, meant when he, having lost four of his children, wrote,

> "When peace like a river attendeth my way,
> When sorrows like sea billows roll,
> Whatever my lot, Thou hast taught me to say,
> It is well, it is well with my soul."

After this five-day period of chemotherapy, Andrew was allowed to go home to Coffs Harbour. Andrew's friend, Lisa, went home also.

Andrew was well enough after a few days to go back to school. However, he was there for only a short time, because, after a month, he was due for his next major course of chemotherapy in Sydney. This time he was placed in the Oncology Ward in the care of a very pleasant young man by the name of Dr. Stewart Kellie.

Andrew had not long been settled into his private room, when a nurse asked him a question. "Andrew, would you mind sharing your room with a girl?"

"Who's the girl?" Andrew asked.

"It's Lisa Augustine," she replied.

"Oh yes!" said Andrew excitedly, "I'd love to share my room with Lisa!"

The two children were to become close friends. I too formed a close friendship with Lisa's parents, Steele and Joanna. When this particular segment of chemotherapy was completed, at the end of that week, they invited Andrew and myself to visit them in their waterfront home in the Sydney suburb of Balmain. This was very convenient for us, since Sandra and her husband, Peter, also lived in Balmain and they had invited Andrew and myself to stay with them for the weekend.

The Augustines lived in a two-storied house with a glorious view of Sydney Harbour and its famous bridge. As we all chatted together over a cup of tea, Steele, who was a member of the Balmain Rugby League Club, leaned across to Andrew and, tapping Andrew's knee with his fist said, "Hey, how would you like to go to a big football match with your Dad this Saturday?"

"Oh, that'd be great!" he replied.

Andrew was a fan of the famous Queensland player, Wally Lewis, of the Gold Coast Seagulls. But he'd never been to a big match, and was elated at the prospect.

The stadium was packed out when we arrived there that Saturday afternoon. However, since we were to be treated as very important guests, we did not have to line up for tickets. We simply gave our names at the entrance and were ushered to specially reserved seats. Steele had also arranged for Andrew to be given team socks, a shirt, a team pennant and a variety of stickers.

I had no idea which team was to play against Balmain, until the spectators began to cheer the two teams on to the field. Then to my great surprise, and Andrew's sheer delight, it turned out to be the Gold Coast Seagulls—with none other than Wally Lewis!

The Seagulls had not been performing too well of late and were expected to lose this match. I told Andrew not to cheer too loudly for them, since they were, after all, the opposition and he was a guest of the home team.

Surprisingly, Balmain lost that afternoon to Wally Lewis and his team, the Seagulls. Their defeat was in no way connected, of course, to Andrew's quite disobedient and highly vocal support of the opposition.

Steele, who had grown very fond of Andrew, gave him a special present following this game. It was a football signed by all the players. Steele's signature was there with Lisa's too.

That ball became one of Andrew's most treasured possessions.

Andrew was feeling so much better following that weekend, that I decided to take him back to Coffs Harbour by train. It was a relaxing and enjoyable journey for us both.

We were only an hour or so from home, when we made a brief stop at the country town of Kempsey. While the train was standing at the platform, Andrew asked, "Dad, I need to go to the toilet."

"That's okay, you can go," I said. "You know where it is," and off he went.

A few moments later, I looked up from the book I'd been reading and glanced out of the window.

I was horrified to see Andrew disappearing into the toilet there on the station platform. As far as he was concerned, one toilet was as good as another. But the train was about to pull out and leave him behind. I threw down my book, dashed through the carriage to the door (which mercifully was still open) then, jumped out onto the platform and rushed into the station toilet. I grabbed Andrew by the hand and thrust him back into our carriage, only a second before the guard blew his whistle and the doors closed.

Because of Andrew's treatment program, we made several train journeys to and from Sydney that year; although none of them had quite the excitement of that one.

Sometimes we traveled by car. Occasionally, if Andrew was not well, we went by plane; several times by air ambulance.

In November of that year, 1992, when we arrived at the Oncology Unit, Andrew was disappointed to find that Lisa was not there. I made some inquiries and found that she was at her home in Balmain. She was being home-nursed. She was dying.

As soon as Andrew had finished his week of chemotherapy, I took him to visit Lisa. It was to be the last time he would see her. She died two days later.

Just before Christmas that year, when I was in Sydney again with Andrew, I arranged to visit Steele and Joanna. I knew that they would both be finding it hard to face this Christmas, the first one without their only child, Lisa.

When we arrived at their house, Steele was not yet back from work. As we waited for him to return, Joanna showed us photographs of Lisa; some of them taken just before she died. Andrew looked hard at every picture. Lisa's death had touched him deeply.

Terminally ill children find it difficult, not only to cope with their own plight, but also the plight of others who, like themselves, are likely to die and often do. In a hospital ward, where every child is terminally ill, the likelihood of close friendships being established, only to be sundered by death, is a very real one. Children, who are well, are not usually called on to face the death of their close companions, as terminally ill children are. For all their tender years, incurably ill children are often thrust into the 'front line' of life—and of death. Here they are forced to suffer the anguish that many adults cannot even face. And some of them somehow manage to cope, with extraordinary understanding and compassion. We adults can learn much from such children.

Joanna knew that as Andrew looked at those pictures of her daughter, he shared her sense of loss.

Finally Steele arrived home. He didn't notice us when he first stepped into the living room. He had just opened his mail and was totally pre-occupied with it. He appeared to be very annoyed about one particular letter.

"I'm flying out to Hong Kong tomorrow and...that stupid girl," he fumed, as he looked at the offending letter, "...I told her to book a five-star hotel for me and she's only booked me into a three-star apartment!"

Before he could say another word, Andrew ran to him and said comfortingly, "Steele, God loves you!"

Steele dropped the letter and put his arms around Andrew. "Do you really believe that God loves me?" he asked.

"Of course He does," said Andrew.

Then stepping back and, holding him at arm's length, he looked hard at him, asking, "Do you believe that God is looking after Lisa now?"

"Of course He is," Andrew replied, with disarming simplicity.

Steele continued to look steadily at Andrew, then narrowing his eyes, said, "You know, Andrew, I didn't believe in God before Lisa died. But now that she is gone, I do. I *do* believe there is a God."

Then, closing his eyes, he hugged him and said, "And you are a wonderful boy, Andrew!"

****

In the following year, 1993, our journeys from Coffs Harbour and back continued, most of them by plane. Andrew loved flying. On one of our late afternoon flights, he sat for several minutes with his face close to the window. He was gazing out towards the distant horizon, with its darkly purpling clouds, their ragged outlines brightly silvered by a rapidly setting sun.

"Isn't God a wonderful Creator?" he said pensively.

"Yes, Andrew, He certainly is," I replied, as I looked out on the scene, my face close to his.

"I want to go to Him now," he said quietly.

"But what about me?" I asked.

"You can come too," he said.

"But what about Natasha?"

"She can come as well."

"But Andrew," I said, with a gentle laugh, "Natasha is not quite ready to leave yet."

He thought about this for a moment or two, then said, "Okay, then I'll stay here."

Although Andrew so longed to be with his Lord in Heaven, he also wanted to live with his family, as a Christian, here on earth. His ambivalence was reminiscent of the Apostle Paul, who explained (in Philippians 1:20-24) that he was in two minds about whether he preferred to live on earth *for* Christ or to be in Heaven *with* Christ.

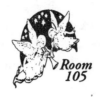

Chapter 29

At Easter, 1993, Andrew was well enough to attend Camp Quality. While he was there, I was able to go to an Easter Camp at Wauchope, where I had been invited as a guest speaker. The people at this camp were all Koreans, so every message had to be translated into Korean. I took the opportunity, while I was there, to ask the lady translator whether she knew the Soo Guen Lee family—Ji-Hye's parents, since I had lost contact with them. I was keen to know, in particular, about Ji-Hye's health. I knew that my chances of locating them were fairly remote, since there were, at that time, about 10,000 Koreans living in Sydney. And, as I'd discovered, when I tried earlier to track them down through the phone directory, the Korean name Lee is about as common as the English name Smith.

The young lady's face broke into a bright oriental smile.

"I know this family!" she said.

"How is their daughter, Ji-Hye?" I asked.

Her expression changed at once.

"Oh...did you not know?"

I feared the worst.

"Ji-Hye died—three years ago."

When I heard this, I felt almost as though I had lost yet another member of my own family. The news also engendered a further reaction in me.

Ji-Hye was dead. Lisa was dead. Would Andrew be next?

I wondered how Ji-Hye's parents had taken the loss—especially Soo Guen, who was still only a young Christian, not long out of Buddhism. I decided to contact them at the earliest opportunity, and this was arranged through my lady interpreter within only two days.

I met Soo Guen Lee at the coffee shop in the Children's Hospital, when Andrew and I were next in Sydney. He was very pleased to see me, as I was him. I was relieved to learn that both he and his wife were continuing on as Christian believers. The loss of their little daughter certainly had not destroyed their faith. However, it had raised (as had Marianne's death for me) many seemingly unanswerable questions—most of them beginning with the word 'why.'

Like me, they had begged God to heal their loved one. Like me, they had been influenced by the guided visualization prayer techniques advocated by their countryman, Dr. Paul Yonggi Cho. And like me, they had been shattered when their loved one died.

I tried my best to share with Soo Guen how I had been deceived by healing doctrines that were really shamanistic counterfeits, and that I had finally begun to realize that, regardless of what I wanted, God could confidently be trusted to do what was right.

As we shared together, I sensed that he was experiencing some other unresolved problems. Although it was now all of three years since his little daughter had died, he and his wife were still grieving deeply. They had not yet been able to summon the resolve to reorganize Ji-Hye's bedroom, but had left it exactly as it was before she died; her furniture, her books, her toys—every item was still in its place.

Soo Guen also shared with me another problem which, he said, had bothered him much. "Brother, Brother," he said with obvious frustration, "I am a Christian, but Buddha is still here," he said, pointing to his left temple, "...here in my mind—*this* side!" Then, indicating his right temple, he said, "*This* side is Jesus!"

He shook his head, as though deeply perplexed, and said, "Big problem, Brother Marcus—Buddha still influencing my life!"

Soo Guen was telling me that, although he had accepted Christ and desired to serve Him, the deeply ingrained teachings of Buddha were still exercising control over his thinking and behavior. It was painfully obvious that my friend was finding it hard to shake off his Buddhist past.

I had long wondered whether some Koreans saw the Christian God of the Bible and Buddha as being somewhat compatible. Did they see, I wondered, the two belief systems as being parallels rather than opposites? Perhaps many of them were still grappling with the biblical notion that conversion to Christ involved much more than a change of allegiance; and that when Christ is really Lord, God works a miracle that changes every part of one's life.

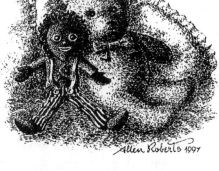

Ji-Hye's Toys

Allen Roberts 1997

"*Therefore, if any man be in Christ, he is a new creature: old things are passed away; behold all things are become new*" (2 Corinthians 5:17).

I later recalled that Dave Hunt and T. A. McMahon, in their book, *The Seduction of Christianity*, had quoted a particularly incisive comment about Korean Christianity in this regard—curiously, from *The Wall Street Journal*:

> "Another trait of Korean Christianity that disturbs some is the tendency, encouraged by prelates like Mr. Cho, to see Christianity as a path to material prosperity. That tendency, critics say, is a residue of shamanism, the native folk religion in Korea and other northeast Asian countries for centuries. In Shamanism, you ask the shaman, a sort of medicine man or woman, to...intercede with the spirits to ensure your health or business success.

> "There is in Korean shamanism a great spirit, above the other spirits, who couldn't be contacted by the shamans. That helped Christianity get off the ground, says David Susan, a Lutheran missionary, because 'when the early Christian missionaries came and said, "There's an almighty God who judges you at your death," Koreans said, "Ah, yes, we've heard of that God before." But in a sense it made Christianity too

> easy for Koreans to accept.... Many Korean Christians
> still consider the gods of shamanism and the God of
> Christianity kindred spirits.'" [1]

"How is Andrew?" Soo Guen Lee asked.

"Until recently, he's been very well. But when he was at Camp Quality, about two weeks ago, he started vomiting again. They're checking that out now. I told him you would be coming to the hospital today. He is looking forward to seeing you."

"Where is he now?"

"He's in gastroenterology. They are running tests on him."

"Can I see him?"

"Sure," I replied, looking at my watch, "his tests will be almost finished now."

We left the shop and walked together down the stairs.

"Do you go to Coffs Harbour again?" he asked.

"Not right away," I explained. "When Andrew's tests are all finished, he'll be going to Disneyland, in the USA, for one week."

"Disneyland!" said Soo Guen with surprise.

"Yes," I continued, "the Guildford Rotary Club is sponsoring six children, with cancer, to go there for a week, with their parents."

"Great!" he smiled, "so you go too!"

"No," I replied. "He'll be going with Beth Rogers, a friend of our family. She has looked after Andrew so wonderfully on so many occasions, I thought it would be nice for her to go with him."

When Soo Guen saw Andrew in his bed, he hugged him and said, "Andrew—you go to Disneyland!"

"Yes, I am going next week!"

Soo Guen took out his wallet and from it removed a 50-dollar bill. He pressed it into Andrew's hand.

"You need some pocket-money!" he whispered.

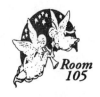

Room 105

Chapter 30

On May 15, 1993, amid much interest from the media, the children in the little Disneyland contingent, with their parents and caretakers (including a doctor and a nurse) flew out from Sydney Airport for Los Angeles.

A few days later, Beth phoned to tell me that Andrew's vomiting had returned. He also had severe pain in his neck. He was too sick to join in all the activities the other children were enjoying so much. His condition was deteriorating.

He was so ill on the return journey that he had to be given oxygen. As soon as the plane landed, he was rushed to the hospital by ambulance.

The radiation, that had been planned before his departure for Disneyland, was begun at once. His condition then improved somewhat and I was able to take him out on a few short visits.

On one occasion, we went, in the ambulance, to visit Claudia and her husband, Warren. On another, we went to the home of Andrew's six-year-old friend, Glenn Smith, who was now off all treatment and was expected to live for only a few more days. As the two boys sat on the couch, holding hands and talking, Glenn's mother Rhonda and I both knew that this would be their last time together. Rhonda could not bear to watch them and went out into the kitchen. I followed her.

She was standing at the kitchen sink with her back to me, looking out through the window.

"God is so cruel!" she said in anger. "Why does He allow children to suffer like this? I can't believe in a loving God anymore."

Then with a note of venom in her voice, she added "I'm finished with God!"

I found it difficult to comfort her. She was in such emotional turmoil, that I knew, from experience, any attempt on my part to explain that God really did care for her, and the boys, would have been premature right then.

Later, perhaps, she might be ready to receive my counsel, but not now.

The next day, it was warm and sunny, so I decided to take Andrew across in his wheelchair to Ronald McDonald House, where I was staying. While we were there, the House Manager, a friendly lady by the name of Helen, noticed that Andrew seemed rather depressed. To help cheer him up, she brought him some paper and colored pencils, then asked him to draw her a picture. He found a black pencil, then rapidly scrawled a number of lines in various directions. When Helen saw this dark, apparently meaningless confusion of scribbled lines, she inquired, "What's that, Andrew?"

"That's how I feel right now," he replied.

Then, handing him another sheet of paper, she said, in an effort to encourage him, "Draw me another picture of how you would like to feel."

Andrew drew a happy, smiling face with bright blue eyes and curly, blonde hair.

"I see," said Helen, as she looked at his drawing, "that is how you'd *like* to feel right now."

"No," said Andrew correcting her, "when I'm in Heaven."

Later that week, Andrew's condition deteriorated again. Claudia and Warren, who were both now working as paramedics, saw that time was running out for him.

"Andy's dying, Dad," Claudia said. "We need to phone Sandra and Natasha right away." They phoned, while I stayed with Andrew.

Natasha, who was in Coffs Harbour, was so distraught when they told her of Andrew's decline, that they offered to drive there and bring her back to Sydney that same day.

They did this, and the following morning saw us all gathered, as a family, around Andrew's bedside: Natasha, Sandra, Claudia and myself. While we were there, the doctor now in charge (Dr. Dalla Pozza) told us that a very recent CAT scan had revealed at last the cause of Andrew's trouble.

The tumor, in his brain stem, had indeed spread—at frightening speed. It was now in the upper part of Andrew's brain, where it could not be irradiated. In fact, there was nothing more that could be done to arrest its growth.

Dr. Dalla Pozza recommended that Andrew remain under his care for another week, during which time he would receive physiotherapy, to remove the congestion that was now seriously constricting his breathing. After this had been done, he saw no reason why Andrew could not be taken back to Coffs Harbour, to spend the remainder of his short life there at home.

This then became the plan, and the next day, Natasha, now a young woman, 19 years of age, went back by train to Coffs Harbour, where she had to move into another apartment that weekend. She looked forward to being with Andrew for his last precious days there.

Andrew was moved into his own room, 105.

As soon as he'd settled in, I sat next to him and said, "Andrew, you will soon be going to Heaven."

Upon hearing these words, he brightened up and said excitedly, squeezing my hand, "When, Dad—tomorrow?"

"It might not be quite as soon as that, Andrew," I told him. "We want to go back to Coffs Harbour first, so you can say good-bye to Natasha and your friends."

Andrew then received a visit from The Starlight Foundation, an organization who try to arrange for terminally ill children to be granted something they have wished for. When Andrew was asked whether there was some place he dearly wished to go, his answer was immediate and predictable.

"Heaven," he replied, thus nominating the one place where no human foundation could arrange to send him. Like Abraham of old, Andrew longed, with the eyes of faith, to go to a city that was not established by human foundations but on heavenly foundations laid by God.

"By faith...(Abraham) looked for a city which hath foundations, whose builder and maker is God" (Hebrews 11:9,10).

We had hoped to get Andrew back to Coffs Harbour by air ambulance on the Friday of that weekend. However, because it was a holiday weekend, we were told that this would not be possible and that we would have to wait until the following Tuesday. I tried to phone Natasha to tell her of this delay and that Andrew's condition had worsened even more, but she had no phone in her new apartment and was unable to be contacted. I prayed that Andrew would not die over the weekend. If this were to happen and Natasha were not to see him beforehand, I knew it would cause problems for her. She was still carrying a great deal of guilt, because she had not said good-bye to her mother, believing, as I had encouraged her to do, that she would be healed.

By Sunday, Andrew was so weak that I was told he would die that day. However, I continued to pray for him. For me, it was not a matter of *whether* Andrew would die, but *when.* Jodi, Andrew's favorite nurse, knew that I wanted to get Andrew back to Coffs Harbour to see his sister and she said to me, "Never fear, Marcus, he'll make it. I'm sure he will!"

At 3:00 p.m. Andrew's school principal suddenly arrived with his wife. They had driven 350 miles from Coffs Harbour to see Andrew and deliver some 30 letters of encouragement from his classmates. Although Andrew was lying there, seemingly oblivious to everything around him, I invited them to come in for a few moments. I was glad I did, for Andrew suddenly opened his eyes, recognized his school principal, and with a cheery smile and a playful hand-slap, greeted him by name. He listened as I read a few of the letters to him, then went back to sleep.

That night, I prayed with him. Then, as he lay there with his oxygen mask on and his eyes closed, I said quietly, "Soon you can go to Jesus."

"I'm lucky," he said, "I'm lucky...I'm lucky...."

He made it through the night and was still lying there peacefully the following afternoon. Just before the nurses on duty were due to leave at four o'clock, they all came in and gathered around me, most of them in tears.

"What a remarkable boy Andrew is," said the nurse in charge. "We have never had a boy like him here before. It is so hard to say good-bye."

One nurse found it so difficult to come to Room 105 and speak to us, that she wrote a short letter. It read:

Dear Marcus and family,

I'm sorry I couldn't say good-bye in person, but I felt that if I saw you before I left, I wouldn't be strong enough to get the words out. I want you to know what an inspiration both you and Andrew have been. Through all his good days and his bad days we've all grown to love him so very much. We will all miss him so much. He has given me so many happy memories.

Your love and strength for Andrew have been an inspiration for us all. No one will miss Andrew like you will, but I know we will all miss him. He will find peace and happiness in his new home.

He is a beautiful boy—a product of his family's love.

Your grief and loss will be felt by us all.

Take care of yourself and your beautiful daughters—keep the memory of their loving brother alive in your hearts forever.

God bless,

Ida.

Claudia, Sandra and their husbands had been wonderfully supportive to me during Andrew's spell in the hospital, and, this night, Claudia insisted that I get some sleep while she kept vigil over her brother.

The next morning Andrew was still with us, and at 6:50 a.m. he was on his way by air ambulance to Coffs Harbour.

A little over an hour later, the plane was taxiing along the runway towards the Coffs Harbour Air Terminal. Standing in front of the entrance, I saw three tall men whom I recognized at once. They were my closest friends, John Smith, Bob Burton and Paul Winterton. I left the plane and walked towards them, my eyes blurred with tears. I fell into their arms weeping, while the paramedics unloaded Andrew and placed him in the waiting ambulance.

Andrew was given a room of his own in the children's ward at the

Coffs Harbour Base Hospital. As soon as he was comfortable, I went to Natasha's apartment. I told her what had transpired since she had left us in Sydney, just four days ago.

She was shocked and angry.

"Why is God doing this to us?" she shouted. "Who is next?"

I gave her some time to come to terms with the situation. Then, when I thought she would be able to cope emotionally with seeing Andrew, drove her to the hospital. I knew she wanted to be alone with him, so I arranged for the visitors to move out and left the two of them together.

Later that day, more of Andrew's school friends came to say good-bye. Andrew assured them that he would soon be seeing the Lord Jesus. Some of his visitors prayed with him. Others sang Christian songs in soft voices. There was a peaceful, almost heavenly atmosphere in the room.

That night, I was told that it would not be long before he died. Sandra, who had flown up from Sydney, sat with me by his bedside, until about 10 o'clock the next morning.

At around that time, when I spoke to Andrew, he opened his eyes and said, "Dad, you are my pal."

These were to be the last words I would ever hear my son speak.

He was unconscious and quite motionless for the next few hours. By mid-afternoon, he was almost in a coma. There were five of us in the room.

I sat next to him, holding his hand and silently praying.

When I opened my eyes, I happened to look up at the clock on the wall. It was 3:57 p.m.

For some reason I cannot yet explain, I felt I should speak to him, although there was now no reason to suppose he could hear me.

"Andrew," I said softly, "those angels you saw, six years ago, are now coming to take you home."

At once, he turned his head, opened his eyes and gazed upwards. It was no blank stare. His blue eyes were bright and focused. There was no doubt about it. Andrew saw something, perhaps someone, none of us could see.

In the next moment, he breathed his final breath, and went to be with his Savior, the Lord Jesus Christ.

Afterword

For God to give His only Son to die for the sins of mankind, must
have brought Him unfathomable pain. In having to let my son
go, I had experienced, as a father, something of that pain also. And
because Jesus' death on the cross was not in vain, so too, the death of
Andrew, as one who had trusted Him, was not in vain either. Jesus'
death was the greatest victory of all history, because He conquered
death, that we might have eternal life. I remember Andrew saying to
a doctor one day, "Jesus conquered death." Because he accepted and
believed this with all his heart, he had no fear of physical death. And
now, at last, he was experiencing the heavenly angelic realm he had
once glimpsed; the dwelling place where there is neither death, nor
pain, nor tears—but only joy unspeakable

When I left the hospital that afternoon, it was already dark, but
inside, I felt a great peace and a quiet satisfaction that now Andrew
was finally in Heaven; the place he had so often designated as his
home.

Andrew's funeral was held in the Coffs Harbour Baptist Church,
where his mother's service had been held, some five years earlier. More
than 500 people attended. The service was shared by ministers from
a number of churches in which Andrew and our family had been
involved. One of those ministers, John Thornton, invited the congregation to do something that is rarely done at a funeral. He asked
them to stand and applaud Andrew for having graduated, by God's

grace, from this life to life in Heaven with his Lord.

Andrew's life was short, but in those few years, his influence was greater than that of many who lived much longer than he. The quality of one's influence is not necessarily a function of time. The ministry of the Lord Jesus Christ was the most powerful and productive ever exercised. Yet it was but three years in duration. Andrew's 'ministry' time extended from when he first became ill until his death—a period of seven years. In that time, he touched innumerable people, especially as he was dying. Although he is no longer with us, he continues to speak, as the New Testament book of Hebrews tells, concerning Abel:

"By faith Abel offered God a more excellent sacrifice than Cain, by which he obtained witness that he was righteous...and by it, he being dead yet speaketh" (Hebrews 11:4).

Andrew's body was buried with that of his mother, and so both are united in the grave. But more importantly, they are now united eternally in Christ.

After the funeral, I received many letters from all over Australia and from overseas. Some letters I cherish particularly, since they testify as to how Andrew had enriched and even changed lives.

One of them was sent to me by Nicola, Andrew's first Camp Quality companion, now a medical doctor. Nicola penned her thoughts in a poem.

FOR ANDREW

Your presence will never leave me.

I will hear your feet pattering, whenever rain on a tin roof is falling.

Your smile will rise gloriously with the sun each day and wink with the moon each night.

Forever existing, lighting and touching the silence in my life like your cheerfulness always used to.

I will see your hope on the faces of young children at play.

I will learn from your simplicity.

I will treasure your joy.

I will draw strength from your courage as I climb up this rock-face of life.

I will pause to observe beauty, like you would.
I will miss you.
I will miss you.
Like a whale's flukes silently sinking in peace.
I will remember your death, and how you still swim free beyond our world.
I will share your faith and daily prepare for when we shall meet once more.
Meanwhile, remember I love you.

I was also much encouraged by a letter from Jodi Pasfield, the nurse who was Andrew's favorite when he was in Room 105:

Dearest Marcus:
This letter is to thank you, Marcus, for teaching and helping me beautifully through the death of Andrew. It is not a sad letter, as we know he is so happy in Heaven, and this is very reassuring, although it does not make it easier.

This is a difficult letter to write, but as I do, I find myself laughing and crying about the times Andrew had in our ward, with his infectious smile and his expressions of love for Jesus. Although these stunned us the first time he said them, I soon realized that he was indeed very special and certainly touched my heart.

Both yours and Andrew's love were so exceptionally strong they extended to all around, making it such a privilege and pleasure to know you. You are both an inspiration to me, and your acceptance and honesty about his impending death, helped to ease this transition. As Andrew was so courageous and eager to go to Heaven, to his mother, there was often a strong calming presence in that Room 105, during those last days.

You have no idea how hard I prayed and urged him to hold on 'til he got home (I knew he would), so your whole family and friends could be there to support you after his death. I wish I could have helped more. Although there were many tears shed saying good-bye, the inner beauty and harmony of you both helped me, as you all were so much at peace with the situation.

Marcus, you and Andrew were both special to me. You taught me so much about life and love and reconfirmed my faith in God, as I laughed and cried my way through his care. Andrew said the angels were too beautiful to describe, and so too are the 'gifts' you and your family have given me during that short month.

Unfortunately Julianna and I were unable to attend the funeral, as all flights were booked up, and I am so, so sorry, but our love and prayers were with you. We are having a service at 1:30 p.m on Monday.

Thank you for everything, and please send me your address, as I would love to call on you. I may be in the area in August.

It seems to me that Andrew's physical affliction, like that of the man who was born blind, was divinely permitted, so that *"the works of God should be made manifest in him"* (John 9:3).

Love always,
Jodi Pasfield.

There are some who think that God is to be blamed for suffering and death. But the Bible teaches, that at the time of creation, suffering and death were not on God's agenda. These things were the terrible result of man's rebellion and sin against a righteous God.

"Wherefore, as by one man, sin entered into the world, and death by sin; and so death passed upon all men, for that all have sinned" (Romans 5:12).

Others claim that an all-powerful God who allows suffering and death to continue, must be heartless and cruel. They fail to recognize the Bible's teaching that God uses suffering and even death for His own divine purposes.

Although God's ultimate purposes are humanly unknowable, we do know that human affliction is God's means of producing godly character in those who endure such affliction; it is a kind of refining process:

"Behold, I have refined thee, but not with silver; I have chosen thee in the furnace of affliction" (Isaiah 48:10).

Furthermore, we are assured that, *"...all things work together for good to them that love God, to them who are called according to his purpose"* (Romans 8:28).

This means, that when some of these "all things" involve suffering, the Christian believer should accept them as having a positive purpose and outcome—for good. Indeed, our response to them should be more than acceptance. It should be one of thanksgiving

"In everything give thanks; for this is the will of God in Christ Jesus concerning you" (1 Thessalonians 5:18).

For me, this "every thing" included some things that I thought at first I would never be able to endure. I do not understand yet, why they happened to me in particular. But I do know that God wanted to teach me things I could never have learned any other way.

I am now quite certain that God has allowed me to suffer such loss in order *"that I may know Him and the power of his resurrection and the fellowship of his sufferings..."* (Philippians 3:10).

I asked Him, as the Divine Potter, to mold me—and He did so.

I longed to grow and bear fruit for Him—so He pruned me.

My experience has been likened, by some, to that of Job, whose suffering is described in the Old Testament. Like Job, I lost members of my family. Like Job, I lost all my worldly possessions. And through it all, I have begun to understand, in some small measure, what Job meant, when he said of God, *"...though he slay me, yet will I trust in him"* (Job 13:15).

Many, and often, were my times of heartbreaking loneliness. These times would come without warning, triggered by something no one else would notice; a word, a phrase, something Marianne would have loved, a fair-haired boy in the supermarket—about the age that Andrew would have been. Sometimes, the unheralded thought would come, that here was yet another thing my daughters had lost and would never have again, because their mother had left them; a word, a timely hug, a needful loving censure—all things that their father, or friends, could never really replace.

When these thoughts assail me, my solace comes from the fact that my loving Lord is no man's debtor; that He longs to make up the things that His children have lost—and has a whole eternity in which to do it:

"...*as it is written, eye hath not seen, nor ear heard, neither have entered into the heart of man, the things God hath prepared for them that love him. But God hath revealed them unto us by His Spirit: for the Spirit searcheth all things, yea, the deep things of God*" (1 Corinthians 2:9,10).

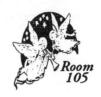

Room
105

End Notes

Chapter 25:

1. Cho, Paul Yonggi, *The Fourth Dimension* (South Plainfield, New Jersey: Bridge Publishing, Inc., 1979), p. 33.
2. Hunt, Dave and McMahon, T.A., *The Seduction of Christianity: Spiritual Discernment in the Last Days* (Eugene, Ore.: Harvest House Publishers, 1985).
3. Ibid., back cover.
4. Ibid.
5. Sanford, Agnes, *The Healing Light* (New York: State Mutual Book & Periodical Service, 1990).
6. Article in *The Advocate*, Coffs Harbour, New South Wales, Australia, December 27, 1986, section 1, p. 1.
7. Schaeffer, Francis, *The Great Evangelical Disaster* (Westchester, Ill.: Crossway Books, 1984), pp. 43, 44.
8. Ibid.

Chapter 29:

1. *The Wall Street Journal*, May 12, 1983, as quoted in Hunt, Dave and McMahon, T.A., op. cit., p. 150.